FAMILY MEDICINE

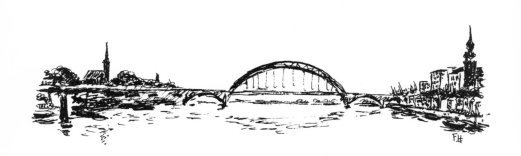

FAMILY MEDICINE

THE MEDICAL LIFE HISTORY OF FAMILIES

by F.J.A. Huygen, M.D.
Professor in the Application of Medicine in the Family

(illustrated by the author)

BRUNNER/MAZEL *Publishers* ● New York

Library of Congress Cataloging in Publication Data

Huygen, F. J. A.
  Family medicine.

  Includes bibliographical references.
  1. Familial diseases—Case studies.
2. Family medicine—Case studies. 3. Family
—Health and hygiene—Netherlands—Nijmegen—
Statistics. 4. Familial diseases—Netherlands—
Nijmegen—Statistics. 5. Family life surveys—
Netherlands—Nijmegen. 6. Health surveys—
Netherlands—Nijmegen. 7. Family medicine.
I. Title. [DNLM: 1. Family practice—Case
studies. 2. Medical history taking. WB 110
H987F 1978a]
RA418.5.F3H89   1982   616   82-12819
ISBN 0-87630-319-X

© 1978 Dekker & Van de Vegt—Nijmegen, The Netherlands

Copyright to the American Edition © 1982 BRUNNER/MAZEL, Inc.,
19 Union Square, New York, New York 10003

MANUFACTURED IN THE UNITED STATES OF AMERICA

Dedicated to the families I had the privilege to serve so long as their personal doctor and whom I came to love.

Foreword to the American Edition

The publication of an American edition of Professor Huygen's classic volume is an occasion for rejoicing. The book has been known to a small number of fortunate readers on this side of the Atlantic since its publication in Holland in 1978, but it has not had the widespread distribution that it deserves and the difficulties of procuring it from abroad have often been frustrating. I have already owned and given away three copies myself.

There are many things to commend about the book. It takes as its subject the medical and psychosocial life history of families, presenting to the reader material collected under an especially fortunate set of circumstances. The population of the area in Holland where the author is a general practitioner stabilized after the Second World War and in the years since then has experienced comparatively little in or out migration. The tradition of relying on the general practitioner to provide the bulk of medical care is strong in the area. At the same time, there is a high level of competence in both the general practitioners and consultant specialists to whom they refer. A stable population in a good relation to its health care practitioners provides an exceptionally favorable observational field for careful, long-term study of the physical and psychological health of families.

Dr. Huygen has taken good advantage of this opportunity. He has come to know these families intimately; he has cared for the family members in their life and death crises and in regard to their apparently trivial and exasperating minor complaints. He has kept meticulous records of all these contacts and has thought deeply about them, looking for *family* patterns of illness.

How does morbidity relate to the family developmental life cycle? Who are the vulnerable members of a family at different points in that cycle? Are there patterns of organ susceptibility to breakdown that are characteristic of a family? These and related questions are explored through the presentation of endlessly fascinating clinical data. An especially important feature of the book is the charting method the author has developed. These genograms graphically spread before us the life events and illness events of each family so that underlying patterns become more evident.

The presentation of this material is especially timely. Family medicine and primary care medicine have grown by leaps and bounds in the United States; at this writing a major new development is taking place. This consists of the rapprochement of systems theory, family therapy, and family medicine. For several decades now, the true synthesis of family and biomedical approaches to human pain and malfunctioning has been sought after. Professor Huygen's book shows us not only that this is necessary, but also how it is possible.

Conceptually, he points us in the direction of a multigenerational biopsychosocial understanding of persons and families—the systemic paradigm in action. Technically, he shows us that family therapists can be integrated into the clinical team and make a measurable contribution to its effectiveness, that family systems therapy can play a major part in facilitating the development of economic and effective institutional solutions to complex problems of health care.

It is not enough to approach these issues with sophisticated theory and shiny new technologies of practice, whether they come from physicians or family therapists. Something more is needed; wisdom, humor and compassion are the qualities I have in mind. They are evident on every page of this book, expressed modestly and with lucidity. What comes through to us as readers is a picture of a careful, thoughtful and highly competent physician, the kind of doctor we would like to be ourselves—or go to for care—keeping detailed and appropriate records and setting them before us comprehensibly and without guile or artifice. The result is a useful and praiseworthy book.

Donald A. Bloch, M.D.,
Director, The Ackerman
Institute for Family Therapy,
New York

Foreword

The catastrophe of World War II proved the watershed for general practice in several European countries. After disruption, destruction and dispersion of families the rebuilding began, the need for personal medical services was again manifest. In many countries the legislation to ensure the availability of medical care as a right regardless of income created a background for such development.

In Holland and Great Britain the reawakening of general practice took similar turns eventually expressed and encouraged through the foundation of Colleges of General Practice. The need for its teaching as an academic discipline and practical skill was recognised and implemented in the two countries almost simultaneously, Utrecht University leading Edinburgh by a short head in the endowment of a Professorial Chair. It was therefore to be expected that books on the content of general practice would begin to appear in both countries.

In a thorough study of doctor and patient, and their mutual trust, Professor Huygen draws upon family groups to whom he is the doctor and true friend. He used his observant eye to draw with, his medical knowledge to draw upon, his feeling for the human situation to draw out. His curiosity and analysis build a picture of a community with its relationships which depict a period of history, geography and human behaviour, complete in itself.

As an intimate recorder of our time he reminds us of a responsibility too few of us in general practice have shouldered. The continuity of medical care, a touchstone of family doctoring is beautifully documented. To the general practitioner reader this book opens the vista of a life-time of work. Professor Huygen's original system of charting medical history against family events demonstrates the opportunity general practice has for organised general observation leading to research. That it is possible to combine a painstaking contribution to knowledge as well as caring for his patients with warmth and humanity throughout the ups and downs of general practice is what this book is about.

William Pickles and Professor Huygen both practised as single-handed practitioners. Whilst Pickles disentangled the infectious diseases, his Dutch successor documented equally painstakingly the complexities of family life and health. The seeds of his notetaking and longitudinal study were sown when, as a young doctor, in 1943, a year before the Arnhem epic took place, he took over this practice.

The description of the team support which includes social workers as well as the priest is compelling in its examples. Furthermore, when this family doctor is integrated with a medical school, he involves its resources; statisticians, psychologists, sociologists, and of course medical students.

Another analyst of general practice, Keith Hodgkin, has taught us the honesty of retrospective outcome assessment, and Professor Huygen follows this humbling practice and his learning while writing:

"Instead of referring them to various specialists (as a way of defence) I should have recognised the family dynamics and should have tried to help with this . . ." "Looking back, I made a serious mistake as we all do. When I saw her again for flat feet I neglected to take her blood pressure. So, in 1960, when re-reading my notes, I went to visit her and found her blood pressure to be 240/140".

It is not only for his medical students in Nijmegen that this book will be of importance, but for all of us who are involved in establishing the content of general practice as a discipline to be taught to medical under and post-graduates.

When machines and laboratories threaten to take over medicine, it is reassuring to read of accurate clinical observations, of clinical judgement, of listening to the patient, of meticulous recording. Thus the role of the general practitioner has been confirmed, and we must thank Professor Huygen for giving us this book from the Netherlands in English.

Dr. E.V. Kuenssberg
President of the Royal College
of General Practitioners

Contents

Foreword to the American Edition   vii

Foreword   ix

Acknowledgements   xiii

Part one   *Case histories* 5

Chapter   I.   A Young Family 7

Chapter   II.   An Older Family 15

Chapter   III.   A Very Young Family 19

Chapter   IV.   Twinned Families 22

Chapter   V.   A Father Dies 35

Chapter   VI.   A Mother Dies 40

Chapter   VII.   Family-patterning in Illness 51

Chapter   VIII.   Problem Families 60

Chapter   IX.   Childless Couples 72

Chapter   X.   Families with a Chronic Patient 81

       1.   A Father with a Chronic Illness 81

       2.   A Mother with a Chronic Illness 83

       3.   A Family with a Handicapped Child 86

       4.   A Family which needed a Chronic Patient 89

Part two   *Family Surveys* 93

Chapter   XI.   A Hundred Younger Families 95

       Introduction 95

       Objects of this study 96

       Results 96

Chapter   XII.   A Hundred Older Families 103

       Methods and material 103

       The comparableness of the younger and older families 103

       A Pilot Study 105

       The hundred younger and older families 106

       Method 111

       Results 111

Chapter XIII.   A Comparison of the 100 family studies with morbidity data of later years 114
Chapter XIV.   A Three-Generation Family Study 123
Chapter XV.   Further Family Investigations 129
Chapter XVI.   Family Therapy 134
Chapter XVII.   Family Medicine 143

Conclusion   152
Appendix   1.   Tables 154
Appendix   2.   Family charts 164

Acknowledgements

This book would never have been written without the continuous support of my faithful secretary Miss Emmy van de Ven, who helped me to collect the data over twenty five years and who did all the typing in her scarce spare time in our busy practice, believing in its value from the beginning.

It would have been less readable if Dr. Robin Steel from Worcester and Mrs. M.F. Geerling-Smith from Amsterdam had not undertaken the task of improving my English, leaving the style and content to be mine. The charts have been conscientiously drawn by Mr. Maas of the Department of Medical Illustrations of the Nijmegen Medical Faculty.

F.J.A. Huygen

Introduction

After more than thirty years of private practice I believe that the time has come to write down some of my observations and experiences. Up till now these have been unpublished although I have often discussed them with students and doctors.

My interest in the medical aspects of the family was aroused in 1960 when I was appointed as a lecturer in what was then called "social medicine of the family". I felt embarrassed at that time, because I did not know what I should lecture about. The head of the department of social medicine, Professor Mertens, warned me not to lecture on clinical family medicine. How right he was in this respect was proved by the fact that even before my first lecture to students a complaint was lodged against me in the Faculty by the Professor of Paediatrics stating that I was lecturing on measles, a subject that belonged to his department. Those were the days when family medicine made its first prudent tentative entrance into the Medical Faculties under the wings of Professors of social medicine (who had often been general practitioners themselves). What should I lecture about without encroaching on the boundaries of the clinical teachers? I soon realised that things would have been much easier if I had been appointed in a branch of science like astronomy with its extensive reference material, whilst there was hardly any literature at that time on "social medicine of the family".

I recalled my personal experiences from memory and realised the precious value of the meticulous notes I had kept since 1943 of all contacts with my patients in their family record file which I inherited from my predecessor in this practice. Perhaps I could use these to tell the students about the medical life history of families, and elaborate on the social implications without coming into conflict with my clinical colleages. Reviewing past contacts with a few families I sought to visualize the form my lectures should take. Beginning with young families I progressed to older couples and from normal families I proceeded to families with a problem (such as death of one of the parents) and thus I concluded with typical problem families.

The presentation of these stories to students proved to be a success. It

1

enabled me to illustrate what was going on in medicine outside the hospital walls and to illuminate the role of the family doctor. Of course I realized the limitations inherent to my anecdotal case study approach. Trying to correct this I elaborated the medical life history of a hundred young and a hundred older families.

Later, an intensive investigation was carried out on a hundred families with the help of a psychologist and a sociologist. Medical students who were specially trained, acted as interviewers. They interviewed the fathers, mothers and children individually and collected a wealth of material in the psychological and sociological fields. These were correlated with the medical data and with the views of the primary health team. Still later psychologists and sociologists of my own department of general practice participated in further investigations. They started with family therapy and I learned much from them. In this book I will follow the same order.

The medical data of the families presented are virtually complete. They comprise all contacts with the family doctor, including those with locum tenens at weekends and holidays, all referrals to specialists and other doctors and all admissions to hospital. I am certain of the details because the recording has been very precise. This practice is the only one in the neighbourhood, and specialists and hospitals in the Netherlands almost always inform the family doctor.

The privilege of being able to gather such a complete and possibly unique set of medical and other data has made me feel under an obligation to publish some of my family histories for the benefit of others. Data like this collected continuously over a considerable period of time becomes more and more rare. People now move more frequently and there is an increasing fragmentation of medical and social care. The community which I serve as a family doctor is however an exceptionally stable one. I now see the third consecutive generation of large families, enabling me to record interesting observations. This population has been so stable because it lives in prosperous villages, the individuals like to remain near their friends and relatives. Many of my families are horticultural farmers, growing flowers and fruit, attached to their land and dividing it among their children who continue to live here and farm with intensified cultivation methods. The city is very near, but the villages are separated from it by a large river whose bridge has not yet spanned this historical barrier.

I hope my observations of medical family life will be of interest to present and future family doctors in different countries, this is why I chose to write in English. Perhaps public health nurses, social workers, clergymen and others who are professionally involved in family life will also be interested. To preserve their historical value, I did not alter anything in my family histories, except that I gave them names of flowers. This implies that perhaps some readers might recognize their personal history and may fear recognition by others. I trust that they will forgive me as it is my intention in publishing these notes to further the well-being of them and others, hoping that lessons can be learnt from these histories by those who have to care for families.

Most of this book is devoted to detailed family case-histories. Chapters XI-XV, however, contain the results of family surveys, while chapter XVI deals with family therapy and chapter XVII with family medicine as an emerging academic discipline.

PART I: CASE HISTORIES

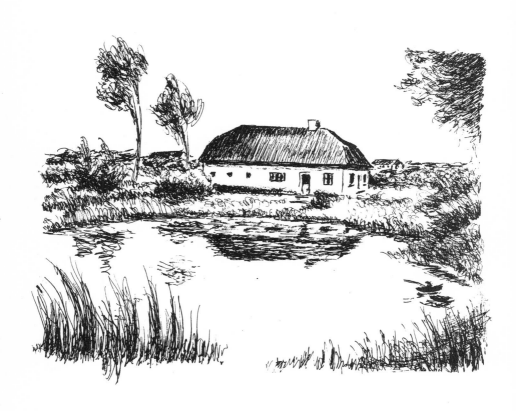

I. A Young Family

At the end of 1944 when the Allied Forces had lost the battle of Arnhem, all women and children had been evacuated from our area. This left only a small bridgehead, northeast of the city of Nijmegen, in danger of being flooded if the dikes were pierced. This the Germans did, putting the thousand remaining civilian men and me as their doctor, literally on an island packed with soldiers and arms. This lasted till the middle of 1945 at which time families were allowed to return.

In 1960 I looked for a family married after the war because I wanted an uninterrupted observation period of a young family. At that time I did not possess a register of dates of marriage of families in the practice, but I recollected that a servant-girl in my house had married shortly after the war and so I took her family as the first in my study. In the survey this family (Azalea) is coded as number 166, but originally it was the first family I studied and I like to retain this historical order.

Betsy married a carpenter in 1947 and went to live with him and his parents in a nice, small whitewashed house on the edge of a fish pond. I expect this house is going to be their property after the death of his parents as this is a usual custom in this neighbourhood. They are very modest in their requests for medical care and this makes it easy to get a view of the medical contacts with the whole family as is shown in chart I.*

---

* These family-charts are gathered together in appendix 2, which can be taken out of the cover of this book in order to enable the reader to have them at hand while reading the medical histories. It is essential to do so to be able fully to follow the histories. The symbols in chart 1 will be used often, so if they are studied carefully it will be easier to understand what is being represented. In the top row the years of observation are indicated. In the left vertical column you see the composition of the family indicated by sex and year of birth of its members. The black Yo-Yo figure before
947 represents the symbol for the marriage. At the bottom of the chart you will find an explanation of the symbols used. The medical contacts with each member of the family are indicated in the horizontal rows at the same level as their year of birth. You will see that there are two rows for the mother; the upper one (with the stork at the beginning) being for the contacts regarding natal care (including ante- and post-), the lower one for the contacts regarding all illness. In the bottom row the total number of contacts for illness with all family members are added per year.

The number of contacts (consultations)

When we study the chart of this three-generation family we see a considerable number of contacts: more than 600, about 500 of them for illness, the latter being almost 18 per year. This gives us an idea about the enormous opportunities for a family doctor to come into contact with family life, to make observations and to exert his influence. No other profession or discipline of medicine has similar opportunities. These contacts were made under varying circumstances, in times of happiness, in disaster or despair, often in critical situations, favouring the possibility of intervention. In these charts I have not entered my contacts with these families in child welfare, but as I run my own "baby-and toddler" clinics, the possibilities of exerting influence on family life are considerably greater even than can be seen in the charts.

Only 1% of the contacts had an emergency character (i.e. were made outside normal working hours or necessitated a break in routine duties), underlining the reasonableness of this family in making medical requests. 3.5% of the contacts required referral to a specialist* and 1% admission to hospital, illustrating the very limited role of hospital medicine in family practice.

It can be seen that eight children were born in the family, all of them at home as was usual in the Netherlands. Birth control was out of the question at that time in this orthodox Roman Catholic family. Things are different nowadays. Almost yearly a child was born, but the last one came 5 years after her predecessor: the end phase of natural fertility.

The average of the annual contacts with the family is 18. This number is attained after a few years and tends to be rather stable, with peaks in the latter part of the observation period. Though it might be expected, there is no definite quantitative correlation between the increase in number of contacts and of family size.

Looking at contacts with individual family members, we see that the mother sought most consultations: almost five a year, not counting the many contacts for maternity care. The end of her fertile period seems to be the time when she needed most medical support. When we realize that many of the contacts with the other members of the family have been initiated by her and took place in her presence, it confirms the observation that the mother is the key figure in family medical care (Kellner 1963). As the years go by her experience increases as is suggested by the observation that the number of contacts with the family doctor required for the young children in their first years of life is evidently considerably less than for the eldest at a comparable age.

The father had a relatively small number of contacts, as had his parents.

---

* Referrals to laboratory and X-ray are excluded.

Patterns of illness

Now let us have a look at the different kinds of illness in this family. To consider these more easily I divided them into some broad categories as indicated in the charts la — lh (appendix 2). Each cross represents a new spell of illness in the category indicated at the top of the chart.

1a. Urogenitary disorders. The mother has been especially liable to these. Her history begins with a cysto-pyelitis in 1947, shortly after marriage. This is often seen and sometimes called "honeymoon cystitis" because association with sexual intercourse is probable. In 1953 she had a spontaneous abortion and again in 1959. In 1960 she had two episodes of urinary infection possibly due to deficient emptying of the bladder caused by a small cystocele. In 1961 she again had a spontaneous abortion and was referred to a gynaecologist for evacuation of the uterus. This was followed by septicaemia, possibly due to cross-infection by her husband or one of her sons who both had boils at the time.

In 1963 she had a severe haemorrhage during the night after her eighth confinement and had to be admitted to hospital for transfusions. In 1966 and 1967 she had menorrhagia, causing anaemia.

It can be seen that all of these disorders of the mother can be brought into relation with her sexual-reproductive function in the family.

Her husband had attacks of kidney stones in 1969 and 1970. In 1970 a stone was seen on the X-ray in the left distal ureter which he passed spontaneously shortly afterwards.

His father passed blood in his urine in 1960, probably due to hypertrophy of the prostate gland. I referred him to an urologist who found an abnormal pyelogram on the right side. The patient refused admission to hospital for operation because he had no further complaints. In 1965 he sustained a urinary infection which responded well to antibiotics.

1b. Upper respiratory tract disorders. These were frequent in the children. Several of them had recurrent bouts of otitis media. The second child suffered from allergic rhinitis in 1967 and 1968. The third child had a mastoiditis in 1953 needing admission to hospital and operation. In the same year his ear started running again leading to adenoidectomy. But in 1969 he appeared to have a chronic otitis media of the same right ear. After tonsillitis in 1970 I again sent him to the E.N.T. specialist, who advised repair of the ear drum. The fifth child also had recurrent otitis media even after tonsillectomy and adenoidectomy, while the last two children also suffered from ear and throat infections.

1c. Lower respiratory tract disorders. Lower respiratory tract infections are specially prevalent in young children but they are also common in old people. The grandfather had several attacks of bronchitis. After the last one in 1969 he suddenly developed congestive heart failure and died.

Interesting from an epidemiological point of view are the facts that in 1952 both grandfather and grandmother were ill with the typical clinical picture of influenza, as were in 1960 husband and wife; yet in both instances the rest of the family escaped from this infection. In my experience children seem to be relatively resistent to influenza virus-infection.

1d. Infectious diseases. In this family my help was only called in for measles in '56, '61 and '68 and for mumps in '72. The chart gives a typical picture of the family epidemiology of measles: it occurs in waves with an interval of several years. Each time all those who have not been in contact with the previous epidemic fall ill.

1e. Cutaneous and mucosal disorders. When I chose this family I supposed it to be quite unremarkable, but when I studied the history I realized that they showed an interesting phenomenon, an unusual liability to skin disorders. Five of the children have had serious trouble with infantile eczema, the third one had to be admitted to hospital for this. Recurrent secondary infections of this eczema gave rise to family epidemics of skin infections including impetigo and boils. The father's small lacerations at work became infected from his children, so that he often presented with cellulitis and lymphangitis. The chart shows these family epidemics. It is known that in some families skin infections can smoulder for years and years. The thousand family study of New Castle upon Tyne (Spence e.a. 1954) has described this and our family is a typical example. I do not think that the explanation would be due to low hygienic standards as in my opinion these were satisfactory. This family demonstrates the far reaching influence of constitution. It is a perfect example of what has been described by Czerny (1913) as "exudative diathesis": a predisposition of skin and mucous membranes to react with exudation, irritation and infections, to all kind of stimuli and of lymphoid tissue to react with hyperplasia. This explains the recurrent ear-nose-and throat trouble of these children and their bronchitic attacks. As described by Czerny, most of them were "white, fat and puffy", yet one of this family was extremely thin and would not grow. The mother developed gross obesity when she was fifty; but I think the father was the carrier of the trait as in later years he often came because of his itching perianal eczema. The recurrent wax in his ears (which his children frequently also had) fits well into the picture as do his kidney stones. The bronchitis of his father had a definite component of bronchospasm and his mother had gallstones.

It is interesting (as regards the skin) to note that warts were unusually frequent in this family, not only with the children but also with the father and his mother. The latter had several on her face, one of them at last developing into a classical basal cell carcinoma for which she was treated by the dermatologist and the plastic surgeon.

In my family studies I became impressed by the importance of constitutional and hereditary factors in common diseases. This is a neglected subject in modern literature, so perhaps it has to be rediscovered and elaborated by family doctors with long standing experience in static populations by careful recording over many years.

1f. Gastro-intestinal disorders were very frequent in this family. Of course several children were infected with threadworms as this is inevitable and there were several outbreaks of gastro-enteritis. Grandmother had gallstone troubles, developing severe jaundice, but she refused operation.

1g. Accidents. The chart shows that boys were more liable to these especially when they grew older. Father's accidents were always connected with his work.

1h. Nervous and functional disorders. Let me first explain that the diagnostic criteria for this are twofold: negative and positive. There must be no evidence of organic pathology to explain the complaints (negative) and there has to be positive evidence or strong suggestion of a psychological explanation. I did not, for example, include in this category the low back pains of the mother which she displayed in 1965 after her father died (though it seems likely that her grief at that time played a role in her symptoms) because she went on to develop the classical clinical picture of a prolapsed disc, which was afterwards confirmed by X-ray.

The chart gives a good picture of the incidence of nervous troubles in a normal family: they are more frequent in the mother, especially in middle age. They occur frequently in the children when they enter the outside world and try to release themselves from their family, especially the girls when they are about to marry.

In the following chapters of this book, when we come to problem families, we will see different pictures.

The symptoms of the mother — nervousness, sleep disturbances — could in every instance be related to family problems. In 1954 her husband had to go on shift work and had difficulties in adapting to this. As a result he was irritable and tense at home. In 1959 he had disagreements with his boss which resulted in palpitations and nervousness for which he later came to my surgery. In both cases the symptoms of the wife mirrored the effect of family interactions, resulting in consultations with the family doctor. In 1970 and later there was tension between parents and children resulting from the generation gap and again the mother translated this into somatic symptoms presented to the doctor. In the last years the father was threatened by dismissal due to socio-economic problems in the building trade.

He was complaining of low back pains for which no organic cause could be established and he was not able to work for more than 50% of his usual capacity. When this had lasted about a year he was threatened to be declared officially unfit for normal work and to be put on a pension. At that time, at the end of the observation period of chart I, I was preparing a symposium on low back pain for general practitioners, with the purpose of illustrating the complex origins of this symptom. Needing a case history as an introduction, I invited Mr. Azalea to the television studio of the university and we recorded this interview in which I tried to find out what was hampering him. It transpired that when he was put back in his working position by a new boss, he felt humiliated and unfairly treated, since no one had told him the reason for his demotion. In the course of our interview, repressed emotions of this visibly depressed man came to the surface and were ventilated. He had not been able to do this before, not even with his wife.

The videotape recording of this interview has been used by the teacher in medical psychology at the symposium and several times afterwards in lectures to students in order to illustrate the dynamics of interviewing technics. I was proud to be able to add that Mr. Azalea soon afterwards recovered completely and resumed full work. I never saw him again in my surgery in the years after this long interview. My pride recently assumed more realistic proportions when I learned from Mrs. Azalea in 1977 that soon after our interview in 1974 her husband got back his former boss, who restored him to his appropiate rank.

The second son of Mr. Azalea had headaches in 1961 which could be related to school problems. The third child started to wet his bed again after the birth of his younger brother in 1954, as did the eldest daughter in 1971, when she was about to marry, whilst emotionally not yet ready for this step.

All this illustrates, I think, the opportunities of a general practitioner for observing and functioning as a doctor to the family. Not all categories of diseases are shown in the charts of this family. Some are omitted, like locomotor- and cardiovascular disorders, because their prevalence was too low. I must, however, mention the fact that the mother suffered a lot from varicose veins, giving rise to recurrent thrombophlebitis, especially in her lying-in periods, and later to several varicose ulcers, which took months to heal. That gives us another example of the evident relation of the diseases of this mother with her reproductive function.

Taking all in all we can say, as I did to myself after studying this first family, that it is worth while trying to look at a family not as a collection of individuals, but as a living and developing unit of interdependent members, sharing common internal and external conditions and showing interactions, reflecting in their medical life history as witnessed by a family doctor.

References:
Czerny, u.Keller (1913), Handbuch II.
Kellner, R. (1963), Family Ill Health, Mind and Medicine monographs, no. 4 London.
Spence, J., W.S. Walton, F.J.W. Miller and I.D.M. Court (1954), A Thousand families in New Castle upon Tyne, Oxford University Press, London.

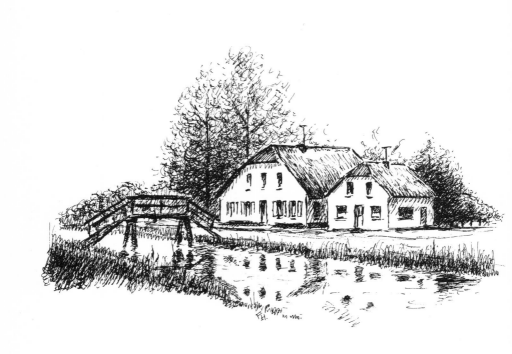

II. An Older Family

After having studied some young families I realized that as a general practitioner you have less contact with families after the children grow up. They require less visiting for childhood infections and there is even a risk of losing contact with the family although its members are occasionally seen in the surgery. So in 1960 I decided to study an older family with adolescent children, with whom I had less contact. I selected the very first suitable family whose house I passed in the street when I started my next daily visiting round. The scrutiny of the notes of this family taught me a lot which I will describe both in this chapter, together with the follow up of this family in their later years. (see chart 2, appendix 2, Family Begonia Sr.). Mr. Begonia Sr. was a nursery man with a large household consisting of Mrs. Begonia, 12 children and his old mother. She had an atrial fibrillation and took digitalis, so, as a young doctor, I did as my predecessor had done and visited her regularly. In the spring of 1944 I ceased the visits as I found the same chats boring and the patient medically uninteresting since she had no complaints. Besides these patients were not insured and thus had to pay for each visit. But some months later she was found dead in her bed and I learnt from the family that she had had oedema of her legs in her last weeks. So after all, I think my predecessor was correct in regularly visiting his old patients, as they are not inclined to call the doctor readily.

When we look at the chart of this family we see that the 12 children were born at regular intervals, except the last one, who came after an interval of seven years, when her mother was 48 years old. It was still then the time of the large family which has definitely ended now in my practice and country. A child born in 1937 with a hydrocephalus who died in 1939 is not included. Besides these 13 children this mother had three spontaneous abortions.

This family was abroad in the evacuation period. We see that the children started to leave the family, one after the other when they were in their twenties, to marry and begin families of their own. We are confronted with the involution-phase of the family. The eldest daughter who stayed at home is a cretin and used to be quiet when all was going well in the family, but started to be very difficult and to demand medical attention when the mother became seriously ill, mimicking her ailments and taking to bed like mother.

This large family is also very reasonable in its demands for medical care and the number of consultations diminished once the small children grew up. In retrospect, it is easy to understand why I selected this family for study in 1960, seeing that I had then had only occasional contact with a few of them in the previous years. The demands for medical care seem to have been even less for girls than for boys. This difference on investigation appears to be due to the higher incidence of accidents in boys. In the involution-phase of the family we see the total number of contacts going up again, which could be noticed also in the first family.

The mother is again the one who needed most medical attention as we also saw in the young family. About the mother I have more to tell later, but first let us look at the medical history of the father. As in the young family of the first chapter his ailments can almost always be related to his work: dermatitis due to contact with primroses, ringworm due to contact with cattle, prepatellar bursitis due to kneeling and small accidents. In later years he became too fat and his blood pressure needed treatment.

Upon reviewing my notes in 1960 I found the mother's medical history very instructive. Her blood pressure was normal in the 1943 pregnancy, after which confinement she had a severe haemorrhage. In 1944 I found a reading of 160/110 with albuminuria, but a normal urine and blood pressure a few weeks later. In 1946 she had a classical lobar pneumonia (as I observed later this tends to occur particularly often in large families) and in 1947 gallstones. In her last pregnancy in 1953 the blood pressure rose to 200/110 in the beginning, but with rest and saltfree diet fell to normal 120/80 in the second half of the pregnancy. At a later routine visit post partum I recorded 170/100 and some albuminuria. I neglected to take her blood pressure when I saw her later for flat feet and Eustachian tube catarrh. So after re-reading my notes in 1960 I went to visit her and found that she then had definite hypertension, the pressure being 240/140, and it appeared on direct questioning that she also had the typical symptoms of angina pectoris. I tried to keep her under regular supervision after that but she tended to default from treatment. It struck me that several of her ailments could be found also in the notes of her children, like recurrent catarrh of the Eustachian tube, postural symptoms due to flat feet and wax in the ear. One of her sons also had hypertension and when I started to check up on her brothers and sisters in the practice, after my experience with her, I found that three of her sisters and one of her brothers had hypertension whilst I heard that a fourth sister living elsewhere was also being treated for high blood pressure. Two of her sisters had gallstones as well and once again I was impressed by the importance of heredity in family medicine.

It was possible to reduce her hypertension and treat her angina reasonably well in the following years, but in 1965 she developed a severe agitated depression. At first I stopped her reserpine medication thinking this to be the cause, but after some time it became apparent to me that the real cause was to be found in the marriage of both her eldest two sons and her fifth daughter. She was very much tied to her children and could not do without them, this being especially so with her second son, of whom I will tell more later. This whole family has always been very closely knit and I think that the term of a symbiotic family used in family dynamics is highly applicable in this case. Each needed the other, which is still so, everybody returning home when one of its members becomes ill.

In the treatment of this mother, the excessive anxiety of her husband and children really was a nuisance; sometimes I had to chase them away from her bed. She was so afraid of dying and her somatic complaints were so impressive that in May 1965 I asked the cardiologist to visit her with me but there appeared to be no signs of a coronary infarction. In November of the same year galloprhythm could be heard, her heart was enlarged and on taking her blood pressure, she had pulsus alternans — by this time a large infarction of the anterior wall was evident on the ECG taken by the consultant cardiologist. In the spring of 1966 a second, this time smaller infarction appeared, and in the autumn of that year she developed diabetes, combined with chronic pyelonephritis. In 1967 and 1968 she had remarkebly little discomfort but just before Christmas 1968 she suddenly dropped dead in the hall. She was 63 years old then and her death was a shattering blow to her family.

In the chapter on twinned families of this book I will go into the tragic story of two of her brothers, who also became depressed and I can also add that one of her sisters afterwards had a chronic pyelonephritis, angina pectoris and a very severe coronary infarction, whilst another sister had severe endogenous depressions. The importance of genetics in family medicine has been illustrated in a dramatic way in the follow up of this mother's personal and family history.

Returning to the second son of this family in 1960 when I was studying the medical history of his family, it struck me that he had had three rather serious accidents in 1959 in a very short space of time and when I saw him again (for wax in the ear then) I asked him whether he possibly could have any problems. He denied this vigourously, but in early 1961 I was phoned by a psychologist whom he had contacted in his military service telling me that there appeared indeed to be a serious problem. The son had been engaged to a pleasant girl for five years, but in the last year he started to accuse this girl of having had sexual contact with someone else. He only wanted to marry a girl who was a chaste virgin although at the same time he was having intercourse with her. The psychologist had the impression that this strange and nervous boy was looking for an excuse to break his engagement. A series of interviews with him did not produce any results. The psychologist thought further psychiatric treatment was indicated, so I referred the boy, but as I never received a report, perhaps he did not go. When I next saw him in 1962 he had a tonsillitis with dramatic symptoms. He then told me that he had been engaged for seven years and that the house and nursery of his father were already divided between him and his brother, but he could not definitely make up his mind to marry. I noted my impression of a very tense and nervous, stammering and explosive boy. I saw him afterwards for erysipelas and other septic skin diseases, but this worry evidently lasted till the end of 1965 at which time he eventually got married. The severe depression of his mother at the same time could now be seen by me in a different light. He did not move far away for he built a house next to his father's. Eventually he married the girl and I came to agree with the psychologist's view of her pleasant character when I got to know her during her pregnancies. They have been married for ten years now, but he still has breakfast, coffee and tea in his parents house. So although he got married he has not left his family.

After his marriage, his youngest brother lives with his wife and children in the father's house where the eldest and youngest sister also resided.

And so the most important lesson I learnt from studying this older family is the discovery that the family seems to have an inherent tendency to stay intact and keep together, to continue its existence and that strong forces are mobilized when its bonds are threatened.

III. A Very Young Family

The older family, described in chapter II, has almost ceased to exist as a family and the young family with whom I started this book is nearly an old family now. Time and society have changed since they began their history. Has the medical life also changed?

More than 150 of the children born in the hundred older families of chapter XII have stayed in my practice after they married and so started a new family. Some dozen of them married a spouse also descended from one of the other older families studied. Mr. Begonia jr. is one of them; he is the eldest son of the family described in chapter II and he married the youngest daughter of family Fuchsia in chapter V.

When we look at the chart of this very young family (chart 3, appendix 2) and compare it with those of their parents, we see both similarities and differences. Like his father, Mr. Begonia jr. does not seek medical advice often. He also is an independent nursery man farmer and does not have the time to be ill. He has hypertension as had his mother and his father, but the high values 180/120 in this young man carry far more serious risks with them. Yet, just as his parents, he defaults from treatment and follow up. His renal functions, fundus and electrocardiogram are still normal and the serum lipids are not elevated, but, thinking of his mother's family, I fear that his life expectation is not a very long one. In 1974 he had renal colic on the left side, passing a stone in his urine shortly afterwards, but X rays showed that he still has a kidneystone on the right. As I recorded in chapter II, one of his mother's brothers also had renal calculi.

Mrs. Begonia jr has always been nervous and tense. She was so as a girl and has remained so. It surprised me that she did not come more often with her worries, but in the first years of her marriage she sought only maternity care. In her first delivery she surprised me with a breech delivery, but with a large episiotomy all went well. Her second child had to be operated on for ileus due to a Meckel's diverticulum.

After a few years Mrs. Begonia jr. started to worry about her children, fearing that they did not eat enough, that their tonsils were too large, that they cried too much and could not sleep. It was evident that she could hardly cope with three children, while her mother did not have nearly as many difficulties with five.

These three children have been carefully planned with an interval of two years between them and the third will be the last one. The most important difference in medical history between this very young family and the older one I think, lies in its span of births. This used to be very long, fifteen years or more in these Roman Catholic families, and now it is shortened to four or less. This couple has been using birth control since the birth of their first child. At first they used the rhythm method, later sheaths, oral contraceptives and in 1972 the husband was sterilized. Yet they are not really a modern family to whom the need of birth control is self-evident and who start with this long before marriage. They have had problems in adjusting to the change of mores. No one was to know that they used the pill and the pill was accused of all sorts of side-effects such as headaches or nervousness.

Mrs. Begonia jr. developed a prolapse as her mother did. She, too, did not want an operation. A lot of worries about her pessary were due to her problems about birth control, but now that her husband has been sterilized these worries have disappeared. He had a difficult time when his mother died.

This is a family in cultural transition. They had to make a break with family traditions, but seem now to have adjusted to this. Apart from the shortening of the span of births, the medical history of this family does not seem to differ much from those of their parents. Counted per child they ask more frequently for advice about health and rearing problems, but the children's diseases are the same as they used to be. As in the older families we see the number of consultations for the children lessen as they grow up, and again the mother seems to have learned from the care of her first child.

There is however one important difference in the health care of this family, that cannot be seen in the chart. Almost all contacts took place in my consulting room, I visited this family only on a few occasions. In the last years house visits are becoming rare mainly due to increased car ownership. The transfer of contacts from the patient's home to the doctor's consulting room — a general phenomenon in the western world — has certain advantages technically, but disadvantages in the psychological and social field, fields which are important in the development of family medicine. The opportunity to meet and observe the family as a whole, to see where it lives and how it interacts, is diminished. I think this is a serious loss, endangering a general practitioner's chances of developing a fuller comprehensive knowledge of the families in his practice in their own homes.

IV. Twinned Families

After the elaboration and study of the medical life history of some dozen families I came to the conclusion that considerable differences existed between them. Some asked for a lot and others for only a little medical help. The spectrum of diseases differed also from family to family, some having many accidents, nervous or respiratory disorders and others less of these, but showing more cutaneous or gastro-intestinal disorders. I asked myself whether it would be possible to investigate these differences. There were many variables to be reckoned with. I had found plenty of evidence that heridity was very important but what of the role of external circumstances?

Every family can be regarded as a unit of its own, with its own composition and character, and just like people, there cannot exist two identical families. But in my practice there happened to be several "twinned families" by which I mean; two brothers who married two sisters. There are at least twenty of such twinned families in the practice and I chose two of these at random, taking into account that the social condition had also to be similar. I scrutinized my notes of these families.

A.   Family 27 and 28 live under the same roof, each occupying half of a semi detached house. Although in reality they share the same surname, I shall call them Cyclamen and Cactus to distinguish them easily. The fathers are brothers and the mothers are sisters. They differ in age, though not very much. The marriage of family Cactus took place in 1935 and of family Cyclamen in 1944. Both couples are of orthodox Roman Catholic religion; family Cactus had 8, and family Cyclamen 11 children. Both fathers are skilled labourers; Mr. Cactus being a stoker and Mr. Cyclamen a cranedriver. Both are mentally stable.

When we compare the diagram of the contacts with these two families we see several differences (chart 4 and 5, appendix 2). Family Cactus has always been much more ready to bring its problems to the doctor. The differences in the total numbers of contacts with the family doctor between the two families over the years make this very evident, taking into account that family Cyclamen was larger. All members of family Cactus have continually been translating their problems and tensions into somatic symptoms, stubbornly believing they had all sorts of organic diseases and demanding referral to specialists.

The medical history of the Cactus family began in 1943 when I took over the practice. The Cyclamen family came in 1952 when they moved in from a neighbouring village. The old parents of the brothers, who lived next door to the Cactus family, needed to be looked after. Grandfather had had a cerebrovascular accident and was demented. Mrs. Cyclamen took care of him for five years and then nursed her mother-in-law who died after suffering a stroke. We can see that Mrs. Cyclamen lost a child in 1954. This boy had been born with Sturge-Weber's disease; he showed ugly haemangiomas on his face and left arm (which was considerably shorter than his right), was a little backward and had convulsions frequently, probably due to cerebral haemangiomas. His mother kept him at home as

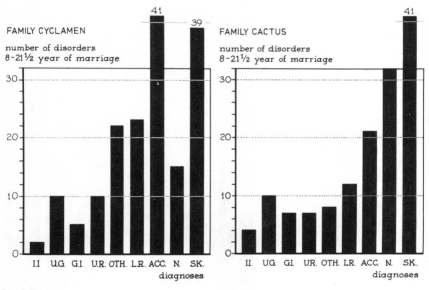

Fig. 1

I.I.   = INFECTIOUS DISEASES
U.G.   = UROGENITAL DISORDERS
G.I.   = GASTRO-INTESTINAL DISORDERS
U.R.   = UPPER RESPIRATORY DISORDERS
OTH.   = OTHER DISORDERS
L.R.   = LOWER RESPIRATORY DISORDERS
ACC.   = ACCIDENTS
N.   = NERVOUS DISORDERS
SK.   = SKIN DISORDERS

23

long as possible, but at last he had to be admitted to an institution for epileptic children where he developed tuberculosis and died.

Mr. Cactus was almost never ill. He had a boil in 1945, minor accidents in 1962 and 1963 and a very severe concussion combined with fractures in 1968, for which he had to stay six weeks in hospital. In 1970 I saw him once for wax in the ear.

Mr. Cyclamen was frequently ill; in 1952 he had recurrent boils for which he had a course of autovaccine. In 1953 he (not being the stoker brother) had a severe pneumonia with delirium, and had to be admitted to hospital. In 1960 he had a pneumonia again; in 1961 a fracture of his ankle; in 1966 a fracture of his big toe and latterly he has had to be admitted to hospital four times in a coronary unit due to coronary infarction. Of course this has given rise to considerable anxiety in the Cyclamen family. It is

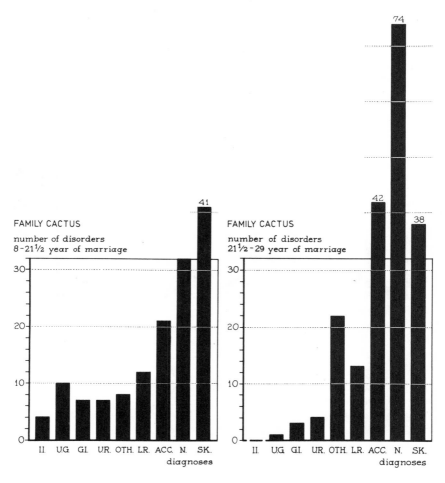

justified in my opinion to conclude from these objective facts that the burden of life to be carried has been much heavier for family Cyclamen than for family Cactus. Still, with the exception of the father, the whole family Cactus was ill much more often. The difference, which must be clear to every observer, is not due to organic disease. On the contrary, there has been more organic disease in family Cyclamen. In the spectrum of diseases of these twinned families there are striking similarities and differences. Similarities are the flat-feet giving rise to postural complaints, the varicose veins, haemorrhoids and skin troubles occurring in both sisters and most of their children, apparently due to common genetic traits. Children in both families have had infantile eczema, and in both families one daughter had very severe acne, probably having something to do with the fact that Mrs. Cactus, like her brother in my practice, has ichthyosis. Mrs. Cactus grew very fat, losing a hopeless struggle against obesity, while Mrs. Cyclamen remained thin, but it was she who developed diabetes in the final years, after having showed transient glucosuria in her last pregnancy. Both sisters had two miscarriages, but it was only Mrs. Cyclamen who had breast abscesses, needing incision, after several of her confinements.

In family Cyclamen the fifth child had severe poliomyelitis and in family Cactus child no. 6 severe meningococcal meningitis. In family Cactus three children had a fracture but in family Cyclamen the children had eight fractures. In both families some of the children stammer or lisp. In 1966 I compared diseases by categories in these twinned families (excluding the common grandparents) by making fig. 1, taking into account only the corresponding years of marriage. Fig. 2 makes it clear that it is necessary indeed to compare similar years of marriage of the families, as definite changes in the spectrum of diseases appear to have taken place in family 28 in a later phase of marriage, nervous disorders sharply rising in incidence. In family 27 there appear to have been more accidents but in family 28 far more nervous disorders. This last trend has continued in the following years as will be very obvious from chart 4 and 5 representing the incidence of nervous disorders in the two families.

As we have seen, in both families nervous problems were brought to the doctor when the children became adolescent. In family Cyclamen only some of the girls were affected but in the Cactus family this phenomenon was much more pronounced where the boys, with the exception of child 3, were also prone to nervous disorders. Child no. 5 had enuresis when he was at home but not when he was in military service. Child no. 4 came, like his mother, so often for his nervous symptoms, that the visits became repetitive and rather tiresome. It is significant to mention, I think, that I was called to his house late one night and found his fiancé having an hysterical fit. She confided she was under treatment by a psychiatrist. I have often wondered over the tendency of neurotic persons to seek partners of a similar personality.

Several of the children of both families are still in the practice now after marriage. The children of family Cactus have grown up to be manifestly neurotic and unhappy, failing in life, while the children of family Cyclamen are sound and happy, most of them climbing to a higher social level than their parents. This difference in outcome between the children of these two families is so very striking that it is almost unbelievable that they descended from twinned families.

In my opinion there is one major factor which explains this difference. The mother in family Cactus has always been a very neurotic woman, as long as I have known her, complaining of nervousness, sleeplessness and all kinds of anxieties, while her sister was much more stable, only having nervous symptoms when the burden she had to carry was very heavy indeed. She, too, had problems when the children wanted to be independent and showed different norms of behaviour than those of her youth; but for her neurotic sister it was absolutely impossible to allow her children to become free.

It is difficult to discover why these two sisters differed so much in their mental health and development. I know only of one reason which I observed which may be relevant.

Mrs. Cactus was the eldest daughter of a mother who was always ill, frequently complaining of headaches and other symptoms which she wanted taken seriously by her whole family. Mrs. Cactus had to take over her family duties when her mother had a stroke. The daughter told me when her sick mother went to sleep, she felt the irresistible urge to have a look at her at least twenty times every hour fearing that she might find her mother dead. I inferred from this story that Mrs. Cactus must have had strong repressed death wishes against her mother. When I cautiously mentioned the possibility of this to her, due to my inexperience at the time, she denied this very vehemently and looked insulted and upset that I should even have had such thought, let alone mentioned it.

However, there is no doubt that the emotional development of Mrs. Cactus has been much more neurotically hampered than that of her younger sister, and that she has conveyed this disorder to her children, giving us a partial clue in our search for the causes of the differences between families in the transmission of illness behaviour.

B.   The second twin family I studied were the families no. 29 and 30 (see chart 6 and 7, appendix 2). I will call them Delphinium and Digitalis. These brothers and sisters were almost of equal age and they married one year after the other. Both families had six children. Both fathers were nursery gardeners and they shared the flower nursery which they had inherited from their father. They did not live in the same house, but in two identical houses next door to each other. Being self-employed, these families were not state-insured and this perhaps played a role in their reluctance to seek medical help. Yet there were very serious illnesses in these families. Mr. Delphinium was much respected in the community, giving sensible advice when asked for his opinion. He was a member of the municipal council and of several local committees. I was called to him urgently in 1946 when he had an epileptic seizure. This was repeated once in 1947 and twice in 1950, always at night, notwithstanding a regular small dose of phenobarbitone, which his wife very conscientiously supervised. He himself thought his fits were of no significance.

In 1951 the ophthalmologist informed me that his vision had worsened rather rapidly. He had found defects in the temporal and inferior quadrants, possibly due to a degenerative process of the optic nerve. Upon his advice I referred Mr. Delphinium to a neurologist who could find nothing other than the reported loss of vision. I think he must have had an arachnoiditis of the optic chiasma. He was given a course of injections with liver extract and vitamin B and his vision gradually improved.

In 1953 he had two further epileptic seizures and in the following years he was seen only occasionally for syringing his ears, because, like his children, the ears were often clogged with wax. I had the impression that this minor ailment, (but for the doctor, gratifying to treat) runs in families. It is perhaps significant to mention that Mr. Delphinium was a brother of Mrs. Begonia sr., whose family (described in chapter II) often had trouble with wax in the ear. He had another tendency in common with his sister. Like her he became severely depressed in 1961 after the death of his wife when he lost his appetite, had insomnia, stayed in bed for several weeks, and neglected his nursery.

His wife was a very nice and sympathetic woman and was seldom ill. In 1953 she had symptoms of gallstone and I regret I did not persuade her more forcefully then to have an operation, because in 1960 when she consulted me again with complaints of weight loss and constipation, I found a mass in the right upper abdomen, which after operation proved to be an anaplastic carcinoma of the gallbladder, the latter containing stones. An anastomosis was established between the gallbladder and the intestine but after the operation she became intensely icteric and died within a month in a hepatic and uramic coma.

There is almost nothing worthwhile to report about the children except for the daughter Alice born in 1939 who had a cardiac murmur from infancy. This was due to mitral stenosis as confirmed by the cardiologist in 1953. She was thought to be too young for operation then. In 1957 Alice had a very serious attack of cardiac asthma with oedema of the lung and when I was called for this on an early Monday morning, finding her exhausted, cyanotic and very dyspnoeic, I remember wondering how could she have waited the whole night before sending for the doctor. She was dangerously ill and disliked the idea of calling the emergency weekend doctor service. After that I referred her again to the cardiologist and this time she was operated on. They found a very narrow opening of 0,8 cm² in a fibrotic valve, but unfortunately, the commissurotomy resulted in mitral insufficiency. For years Alice lived on the verge of congestive failure. I saw her every month to give her an injection of long acting penicillin. In the end of 1962 her heart became enlarged and began to fibrillate and in the beginning of 1963 she had either pneumonia or perhaps a pulmonary embolism. I sent her again to the cardiologist, who admitted her to see if further operation was possible which, alas, it was not. I remember having a serious interview with Alice, when she returned home, about the limitation this meant with her future activities. I was relieved to hear that she was not engaged, but I had to advise her against ever marrying and this was a shock to Alice. Soon she began to run a fever, making me fear the possibility of subacute bacterial endocarditis, which proved to be the case when she was re-admitted to hospital. After a month of searching, the streptococcus viridans was cultured from her blood. She received several intensive courses with antibiotics before she came home, but within three weeks she suddenly became paralysed on the left side of her body, due to cerebral embolism. Alice was very restless and anxious, and I had to visit her frequently, often several times a day. She remained paralysed and she had great difficulty accepting her disability. She really was a very pretty and fine young girl who still expected so much from life. Would she never be able to dance again, she asked me in despair. I remember we had several earnest and deep conversations, and I can still see before me the fine picture of Van Gogh's blossoming peachtree that hung above her bed. In January 1964 she got fever again with signs of a pneumonia — probably due to renewed septic embolism. Alice was desperately ill and refused to fight, as she did not want to go on living with her paralysis. She died on January the eighteenth at the age of 24.

One day in the autumn of 1963 while I was visiting Alice I found her father to be very ill. He ran a high fever and I discovered the signs of a left lower lobe pneumonia. He also had signs of emphysema but I was more alarmed by his appearance as he was very thin and slightly cyanotic. I remember having exchanged a look of understanding, after examining him, with the student who accompanied me, agreeing in the car afterwards that this presentation was highly suspicious of bronchial carcinoma. After his temperature fell with antibiotic treatment, I referred him to the chest physician, who found a destroyed left lung. He advised immediate admission to a chest clinic where the diagnosis of bronchial carcinoma was confirmed and a pneumonectomy performed. He returned home in time to witness the death of his beloved daughter and was severely depressed thereafter managing to hold his own until the autumn of that year, when he started to speak clumsily and to walk unsteadily. I found abnormalities of the pupils and reflexes and consulted the neurologist who advised cyto-

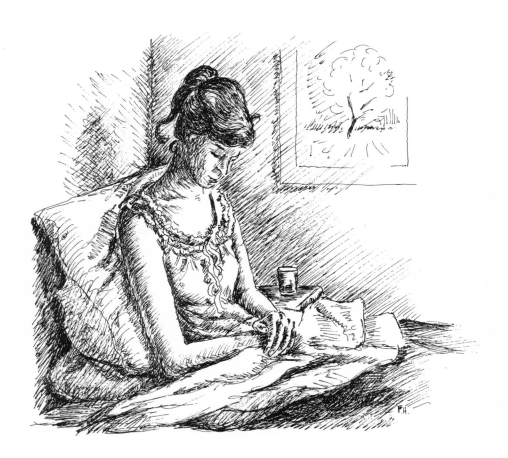

toxic therapy. But his symptoms worsened and he told me himself that he thought he was going to the "eternal hunting fields", which he did on December the fifteenth at the age of 64. On his death certificate I filled in the diagnosis of bronchial carcinoma with cerebral metastasis. The two remaining children married shortly afterwards.

The story of family Digitalis is no less a dramatic one. Mr. Digitalis had a kerion in 1945 and renal stones in 1947. When I referred him to the radiologist, polycystic kidneys were demonstrated on I.V.P. His blood pressure was 140/90 at that time. In 1948 he had a depression which lasted several months. In the following years he had intermittent haematuria and renal colics. In 1958 the diagnosis of chronic bronchitis and emphysema was established and his blood pressure had risen to 220/130, his circulation time being 15 seconds. I attempted to reduce his blood pressure with some success. In 1960 he again became depressed, due to the fact that his favourite daughter had to be admitted to hospital. As in his brother's family this daughter was the fourth child. She was not very pretty, but she resembled her father and they were very close. She started nervous symptoms in 1959, gradually worsening in the autumn of 1960. She was obsessed with weight and dieting, slept badly, kept crying and finally stayed in bed. She had the typical symptoms of a severe depression, but her preoccupation about her thinness was somewhat disturbing to me, even in an infantile girl who had never been away from home.

The psychiatrist who admitted her to hospital, wrote in his discharge letter that he had established the diagnosis of a neurotic depression in a girl with very limited intelligence. He thought that she tried to express her adolescent problems in her longing to put on weight. Her schizoid symptoms disappeared in a few days and he treated her with medicine and a course of insulin. She was much better when she came home at the beginning of 1961. I spoke with her about the possibility of looking for a job, but she stayed at home, helping her father in the nursery. Her mother told me with a laugh that she was a typical father's child. In the spring of 1964, after the tragic death of her niece, she again became depressed and on a Sunday morning, ten minutes after having been lying in bed with her father, something she often did, she was found in the barn, having hanged herself. In retrospect I strongly favor a diagnosis of schizophrenia.

Her father reacted with a severe depression, not responding to anti-depressants and the next year he too suddenly died, probably due to a cerebral haemorrhage or a coronary infarction.

Both father and mother of this family have always been less strong than their brother and sister, not only mentally, but also physically, and their children were less strong in comparison to the children of family Delphinium. Perhaps it is significant to mention that three of these children had cerebral symptoms. In the third child this manifested itself with

FAMILY DELPHINIUM

number of disorders
12½-32^e year of marriage

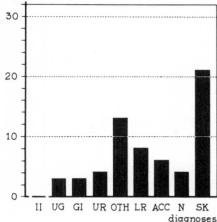

FAMILY DIGITALIS

number of disorders
12½-32^e year of marriage

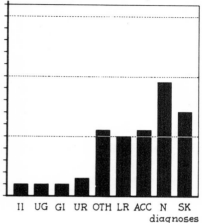

Fig. 3.

I.I.	=	INFECTIOUS DISEASES
U.G.	=	UROGENITAL DISORDERS
G.I.	=	GASTRO-INTESTINAL DISORDERS
U.R.	=	UPPER RESPIRATORY DISORDERS

OTH.	=	OTHER DSORDERS
L.R.	=	LOWER RESPIRATORY DISORDERS
ACC.	=	ACCIDENTS
N.	=	NERVOUS DISORDERS
SK.	=	SKIN DISORDERS

periods of vertigo and vomiting in 1965. In the fifth child, periods of headaches, drowsiness, confusion and diplopia in 1959 made me think of encephalitis which led to hospital admission. Child no. 6 suffered a period of headaches, vomiting and vertigo after his smallpox vaccination in 1962 when he was in military service. This last boy later had many problems, being afraid of marriage and at last selling his father's nursery which he could not manage.

In fig. 3 I compare the spectrum of morbidity in these two families. The differences are not large, except in accidents and nervous disorders as with families 27 and 28. Charts 6 and 7 (appendix 2) show the episodes of nervous disorders in both families. The difference is striking and we can see that it is not due to one or two individuals, but that the nervous disorders are spread over the whole of family no. 30.

Once again we see that the family with the most heavy burden to carry (the death of the mother and the cardiac disease of the daughter) has showed the least nervous problems. As in family 27 the mother of that family had the most stable and harmonious character of the two sisters and I think this is the most important factor in the explanation of the difference between these two families, though in this case there was also a similar difference between the fathers.

31

Scrutinizing my notes I find that Mrs. Digitalis, like her sister, had symptoms in 1963 that perhaps could be attributed to gall stones. When I see her again one of these days I will suggest that she should have an X ray; prevention being better than cure.

When I finished the study of this second pair of twinned families I was impressed by several points; the familial tendency to severe depressions and the apparent liability of the central nervous system of these families to organic and functional disorders. But above all I was not only impressed but even a little depressed by the doom that seemed to have lingered above these twinned families. In both a young girl, the fourth child, favourite of the father, came to die at the same time and both fathers died shortly afterwards. Is fate so inescapable in family medicine?

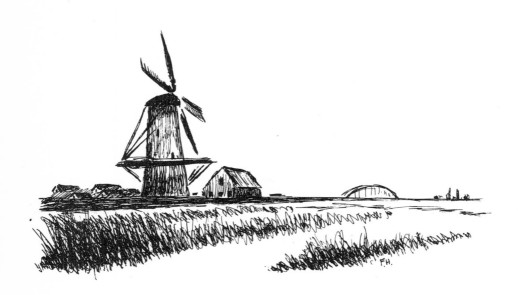

V. A Father Dies

A. Mr. Erica and his wife had three children; a daughter and two sons (chart 8, appendix 2). Their families had lived in our village as farmers and were respected families in this community. When he was a young man he took off to the most luxurious residence of the Netherlands and went into service as the chauffeur of a wealthy noble lady. This was very much against the wishes of his parents and gave rise to a lot of family trouble. They were very glad when at last he returned home and settled down, taking over a flourishing flour mill and bakery in the same quarter of the village where they lived. This neighbourhood seems to be inhabited by one very extensive family and indeed most of the families are more or less related. The area is large, each year it has its own fair, and when the farmers go to the centre of Bridgevillage they speak as though this were a different town.

Although the mill and the bakery trade did not quite suit his taste, as his sons told me later, Mr. Erica worked hard and prospered. He was respected in the whole village and he rendered services to the neighbourhood, for instance he transmitted messages to the doctor, even during the night, as he was one of the first to have a telephone. He was hardly ever ill himself. The first time his wife called me was in November 1949. He ran a fever, and he seemed to have lost some weight, while it had struck his family that his temper was less good than it usually was. I could find nothing abnormal, except albuminuria. His fever soon disappeared, but his usual feeling of well-being did not return, he felt exhausted, listless and he perspired during the night. I had to reconsider my provisional diagnosis of flu and I investigated further. The sedimentation rate of his blood appeared to be 53/93 and, though his stools did not contain occult blood, at the end of the month I palpated a painful lump in his left lower abdomen. Accordingly I sent him to a specialist in internal medicine, who reported on January the 11th, 1950 that he saw an obstruction on the X-ray of his left colon and advised a laparotomy. Mr. Erica did not like this idea and I had to visit him twice before he agreed to be admitted to hospital (for the first time in his life). He proved to be right in his apprehension, for the surgeon found an inoperable carcinoma of his colon, his left ureter being involved in the local mass. He died two days after the operation at the age of 56.

When we look at the diagram of the medical history of his family in order to investigate the impact of this short drama, we do not see spectacular changes after his death. Of course I visited his wife in 1950 to sympathize with her. In the same year I saw the daughter twice for low back pain, and again twice for an exudative tonsillitis. In 1952 she left the family because she was getting married.

In 1951 I got a letter from the medical examination board, telling me that the youngest son was rejected for military service because of his varicose veins and I saw him once in November for a rash on his forearms, perhaps due to contact with flour.

Upon examining the chart it becomes clear, that the medical consultations of the mother began to increase at this time. Studying the content of these contacts several symptom complexes become apparent:
1. a variety of nervous symptoms: nervousness, vague abdominal symptoms, sleep disturbances, an emotional collapse in 1952, overwhelmed by difficulties, dizziness, low back pain etc.
2. varicose veins, haemorrhoids and flat feet gave rise to symptoms not only in her case, but also in both her sons, pointing to some possible hereditary weakness of connective tissue,
3. she was getting fat, reaching a weight of 96 kg while her height is only 167 cm,
4. at the same time her blood pressure rose, needing regular supervision,
5. she complained bitterly about her brachialgia, which incapacitated her,
6. in 1955 she complained of an itching anal dermatitis, but it was only in 1959 that latent diabetes becomes apparent. Her mother also had had diabetes and her sister later developed glucosuria. It seemed to be very difficult for her to diet and in 1965 she had to be admitted to hospital because by neglecting her diet her weight soared,
7. in 1964 she developed uterine prolapse, which was controlled by a pessary and needed changing regularly.
Several of these symptoms can be attributed to her constitution and her age while others are related to her widowhood and weight gain.

The elder son, whom I treated in 1944 for scarlet fever and for cryptorchism and in 1949 (while doing his military service) for an ischio-rectal abscess due to haemorrhoids, was in 1950 released from his military duties to take the place of his father. In 1952 he started to complain about his back, perhaps due to his extreme flat feet, and afterwards of an intractable cough for which no cause could be traced. After a while it became clear to me that he did not like the bakery trade and that he was using his cough (blaming the flour) and other nervous symptoms to escape from his duties without upsetting his mother. In 1955 he worked as a truck driver causing much grief to his mother who regarded this as a social degradation. Later on a compromise was reached when he started a successful driving school. He married in the spring of 1955 but never had children, perhaps due to his undescended testicles as a boy.

The younger son started to have all kinds of nervous symptoms when he was to take over the bakery in 1955. In the beginning of the sixties he helped his brother in his spare time as a driving instructor and had several accidents through inattention. In 1964 I had a long interview with him as he was seriously depressed. He did not know what he was going to do; he did not like the bakery trade either. He firmly believed that his brother was going to invite him in as his partner in the driving school, but quite unexpectedly his brother refused this. This was a shattering blow to the younger son, then 32 years old. What was he going to do now? In church, in the cinema and in company he experienced phobic anxiety and panic. I had a long interview with him and afterwards he appeared to have decided to go into motor trade, first as a driver, but later succeeding in developing a transport business of his own. He married in the autumn of 1966.

Both sons are doing well since they have married and I do not see much of them. Neither of them has shown any further nervous troubles.

The mother has had serious problems finding a new place to settle down after she had to leave the bakery. I still see her regularly for her diabetes and she still complains of all kinds of symptoms; she does not seem to be very happy though she is resigned. She and the younger son have both left their original neighbourhood.

B.   Mr. Fuchsia (see chart 9, appendix 2) lived near Mr. Erica. He and his wife had five children and ran a flower nursery. Mr. Fuchsia too was seldom ill, I saw him before the evacuation period in the war only for small wounds and for an olecranon bursitis. At the end of 1949 he began to complain of fatigue and lack of appetite. I found his blood pressure to be 220/120 with albumen, casts and red blood cells in his urine. His heart was enlarged and there was some pitting oedema in his legs. I referred him to the specialist in internal medicine, who found that his blood urea was 1000 mg%, creatinine clearance being only 27%. Though the fundus showed no retinal changes, the specialist agreed that the diagnosis of malignant hypertension had to be seriously considered. This proved to be the case, his blood pressure going up to 240/170 and his urea clearance falling to 6% in spite of treatment with rest, diet and medicine. In those days we were unable to treat malignant hypertension effectively. It is peculiar that our patient felt very well, he only complained about his tasteless salt and protein free diet which he found abominable. He came to rely heavily upon me during his terminal illness. In 1951 he developed gross oedema, due to hypoproteinemia and had a transient hemiparesis with speech difficulties which disappeared with bedrest. In the beginning of 1952 he suddenly died, probably due to a cerebral haemorrhage. His age then was 58 years.

I had been seeing his wife regularly because she needed a pessary for a vaginal prolapse and she had gallstones, and was unwilling to submit to an operation. She had also several times had transient symptoms of rheumatic disease but it was not she, but her sister, who went on to develop the typical picture of rheumatoid arthritis complete with tendon rupture in her fingers.

One month after the death of her husband Mrs. Fuchsia complained for the first time of angina and in August of 1953 she had a severe anginal episode. There were, however, no definite signs of recent infarction on the electro-cardiogram as recorded by the specialist. As her temperature rose, bedrest was prescribed with anticoagulants. At that time she had already become grossly obese, and she never succeeded in reducing despite dieting. Perhaps she compensated for lack of satisfaction by eating.

In 1955, three years after the loss of her husband, she started to have her first vague nervous complaints, the next year these culminated in an hysterical state with blackouts and later states of excitement. Serious conflicts had arisen between her and her children. She did not allow them any freedom and it is significant that she paid her son, who then ran the nursery, only enough to buy one packet of cigarettes a week. The most controversial point seemed to be her disapproval of her children's proposed fiancés. Sent away to try to find some rest and recuperation, she came back within a few days against advice.

At the same time her children were consulting me for a variety of nervous symptoms which later however subsided. In 1960 the two eldest children married and left the family. The nursery was divided between the son and the son-in-law. A progressive blindness became apparent now in the mother, due to macular degeneration. She had problems with her pessary, losing it again and again and reluctantly deciding to be operated on in 1962. But as so often happens, at least in my experience, within a short time vaginal prolapse symptoms appeared again.

In 1963 she developed congestive cardiac failure, reacting well to digitalis, restriction of salt intake and diuretics. Then in August 1964, while hurrying to catch the bus after doing some shopping in the city, she suddenly collapsed in the street and died at the age of 67, death most probably due to myocardial infarction. She was descended from a large family of 14 children and I have looked after five of her brothers. All of them died of myocardial infarction, three of them having had several attacks. I knew two of her sisters; one died suddenly, the other is crippled by rheumatoid arthritis but she also has the signs and symptoms of coronary insufficiency.

When we look at the charts of the nervous disorders in these two families (chart 8a and 9a, appendix 2) it becomes at once clear that we are not dealing with individual disorders, but with a disorder of the family system. All members were involved at the same time. (Even the resident servant in the baker family, who is not in the chart, showed the same troubles at that time). It is very improbable that these symptoms were due to individual grief and sorrow; in both families the symptoms appeared after a silent period of about two years. In both families there were serious internal tensions and conflicts between mother and children at that time. The mothers tried to take over the roles of their husbands to keep rule and order, thereby creating antagonisms. Perhaps it is significant that both families still had an important socio-economic productive function; they were not only units of living but also units of working. The fathers were not only the head of the family, but at the same time head of the firm. This gave rise to an old-fashioned authoritative patriarchal power structure. It is only in families like this that I can remember having seen similar repercussions after the death of the father. In other families with a less strong power structure, it is my impression that the children, especially the sons, often afterwards fail in society. If the father dies when they are young, the eldest son has the risk of being elevated by his mother to take over the role of supporting her as a (substitute) husband, with serious risks for the son's mental health.

Until now all children (excepting the daughter of family Erica) have remained in my practive after their marriage. (Mrs. Begonia described in chapter III, is a daughter of Mrs. Fuchsia.) All of them are doing well and none of them show any abnormalities. As their family doctor I will have to be on the alert, being on the lookout for diabetes in the Erica children and for cardiovascular disease in the Fuchsia children.

In addition to this, the study of these two family histories, with the father's premature death, has taught me once again that the family must indeed be looked upon as a unit in itself, a unit with its own disorders, diseases and pathogenesis.

VI. A Mother Dies

A.   Mrs. Geranium (see chart 10, appendix 2) was a small, very unattractive woman, with an ugly white sebaceous skin, strong spectacles and a low husky voice. Her family was tuberculoid and that fate ultimately determined her. She was married to a small farmer, whose mother had been admitted to a mental institute for schizophrenia. He had a cold and frigid, old-fashioned personality and in their home there always was an atmosphere of unhealthy gloom

When I was called to this house in the spring of 1943 for the first time, she was in labour with a seventh pregnancy having had no antenatal care. All children had impetigo see chart no. 10a). In that summer she developed a nasty lobar pneumonia with pleural effusion. X-rays taken in convalescence revealed signs of old tuberculous lesions in the apices of both her lungs, so she was kept under regular follow up for this by the chest physician. In 1946, after the birth of her ninth child, the tuberculosis flared up and she was admitted to a cottage hospital where I looked after her. In 1947 she was sufficiently recovered to go home. Now gallstone trouble started but soon she became pregnant again, when tubercle bacilli were found in her urine. Admittance to a sanatorium was arranged after her delivery whilst the baby was sent to relatives. When at last she was admitted, it appeared she was pregnant once again. She was at that stage in a bad state with anemia, gallstones, cholecystitis, tuberculosis of lungs, kidney and bladder. But she improved greatly after a nephrectomy half a year after labour had been induced before term. An artificial pneumothorax was succesful and she appeared on the way to good recovery when, during a refill of her pneumothorax, she suddenly died due to air embolism at the age of 48.

When we look at the chart we see that her family already had begun to disintegrate: the youngest children had been placed elsewhere, but some of them came back after her death. The neighbour looked after child no. 8 for six months and after child no. 10 for 6 years. Afterwards she confided to me she never received a penny for this and that she even had to pay for the milk she bought from Mr. Geranium for his own children! This motherly warm woman never got a word of thanks for all she did.

In the years following nothing striking caught my attention in this family, except that child number 4 had a very severe parathion intoxication in 1955. I was called in the middle of the night; he had been vomiting and was in coma now. He looked very bad, cold and perspiring, deeply unconscious, with pin-point pupils, fibrillating and had generalized clonic contractions. His dirty hands and feet were still coloured yellow by the agricultural poison with which he had been working; he had not even taken the trouble to wash them after his work. He was admitted to hospital and had a very narrow escape from death.

Perhaps it is relevant to mention in the history of this motherless family that three of the sons (child no. 6, 9 and 10) went into a seminary to become priests when they were twelve years old. Only one of them (no. 9) returned afterwards.

It was not until 1960 — ten years after the death of the mother — that I was asked especially to see one of the daughters, Ann (child no. 5). She was then almost twenty years old and was a servant in a household with children. One evening her mistress telephoned me to say that Ann was lost; she had left the house but she had not reached home. During a search next morning she was found in a dry ditch, she was mute and was put in bed. Her mistress asked me to examine her and to have a talk with her. It transpired that Ann had had intercourse with an unknown man (who prudently used a sheath) and that afterwards she did not dare to go home. Talking with her was very difficult, because she gave few answers. Her only complaints were severe headaches, I saw her several times for these. I understood that Ann was in conflict with her stern father, but still more with her eldest sister Martha. Her mistress told me that Ann was forced to rise at four o'clock in the morning, to go and work in a farm elsewhere, from six to eight she had to help at home, then she went to her mistress till 7.30 each evening and after that did farm work again till 11 o'clock at night. She did not get any of her own wages. I consulted a social worker and we decided to go to her father, who worked for someone else, his own small unproductive farm being looked after by the eldest son. I got his consent to let Ann stay day and night with her mistress and family, with whom she had a very good relationship. Her mistress treated her as one of her own children, and the social worker arranged for social activities during her leisure time. But we made a serious mistake. We did not consult Martha, who had taken over the role of the mother, and who had already been giving warning signs in the previous months; dysuria without abnormalities in the urine, dysmenorrhoea and staying in bed without apparent reasons. She came to claim her sister saying that she would go crazy if Ann did not come home. What could somebody else give to Ann that she could not give? The social worker tried in vain to talk with Martha; Martha only wept and screamed. I visited her several times and had long — mostly silent — interviews with her. But I did succeed in establishing some kind of rapport with her. I started by relieving her of several ugly sebaceous cysts and treating her gross acne. Gradually she began to open up, telling me how hurt she was on hearing that Ann disliked her. It appeared that Martha was genuinely concerned and anxious about all the children, but especially worried about the light-heartedness of Ann's character. At the same time some Freudian jealousy became apparent, as her father seemed to prefer Ann, the prettier daughter.

Looking back I must say that Martha was proven right in her worry. Ann managed to contact afterwards all sorts of men and boys of bad repute and did stupid things in her craving for warmth and affection. We invoked the help of a child-guidance clinic when she ran away. Her intellectual capacity seemed to be much lower than expected from her appearance and the impression she made on others. In the following years we held our breath several times, but at last she married a nice boy who gave up his fiancée for her.

In the meantime the youngest daughter Kathleen started running away from home, unable to cope with the tyranny of her overanxious sister Martha. In 1962 I saw Kathleen for severe abdominal pains, when she was helping in the house of a recently delivered neighbour. She rolled to and fro in the new mother's bed and seemed to be in state of fright and hysteria. Examination was almost impossible but her temperature had risen and she had a leucocytosis. So to exclude the possibility of appendicitis I sent Kathleen was of normal intelligence and character, outwardly without the diagnosis of appendicitis but it transpired she had infectious mononu-cleosis, the reaction of Paul-Bunnell going up from 1:28 to 1:64! The surgeon doubted whether this could explain the tummy-aches she kept complaining of after her discharge. The next month Kathleen had a severe exacerbation of her colicky pains, necessitating re-admission. This time the specialist in internal medicine observed her as an in-patient for seven weeks and was unable to find any abnormality, nor could the gynaecolog-ist. Her colic responded immediately to injections of saline-water and so the psychologist was consulted who wrote a long report, stating that Kathleen was of normal intelligence and character, outwardly without apparent emotions, but inwardly full of repressed emotions. He discovered two stress factors: the un-integrated death of her mother, by whom she felt deserted, and the frustrating relationship with her dominant sister Martha. The psychologist thought it probable, that Kathleen's colic pains were provoked by the circumstance that she was helping in a family where a child was born. On the one hand she was confronted with a mother and child relationship, which aggravated the deep loss of her own mother. On the other hand her longing to be independent and to leave home was re-activated, while at the same time she knew she had to go back home again. I think it was not merely coincidental that I found Kathleen in the bed of a recently delivered neighbour, when I was called for the first time.

At the same time I must also say that six months later, when I was called again during the night for her abdominal pains, I again found a raised temperature and that this time after operation on microscopic examination her appendix appeared to be acutely inflamed, with hard faecoliths and scars of previous inflammations! Therefore in retrospect, I think this history is a perfect example of the problems of a family doctor who has to pay due attention to the physical diseases and at the same time to the emotional causes of symptoms of his (or her) patients.

The healing of Kathleen's operation scar gave a lot of trouble, showing signs of recurring infections and forcing me in the end to do a wide excision since I suspected sebaceous lesions similar to those of several of her brothers. But on microscopic examination nothing could be found except foreign body giant-cells. The pathologist suggested in his report the possibility of an artefact due to manipulation by the patient.

The social worker tried to help this family, but it soon became apparent that Martha regarded her as the ally of Ann and her employer. She even refused to help in the work-up of the child-guidance clinic. A second social worker who was working with me in the practice at that time and who had never had any contacts with Ann, was more acceptable. In close co-ordination we succeeded in winning Martha's confidence and in giving her some support in her difficult situation. We encouraged her to widen her interests outside the family and at last we got her so far as to become a hospital nurse and to hand her duty as the caretaker of the family over to Kathleen. Martha became a quite different and happy girl and was successful in her job. Despite the circumstance that Mr. Geranium at this time developed a cavernous tuberculosis of the lung, things went reasonably well with this family.

Mr. Geranium recovered, but he became grossly obese. He is at home now, doing almost nothing except preparing meals, having had a lot of trouble with temporary housekeepers. The youngest daughter Kathleen is happily married, and now has two children of her own. Two sons are still at home: one being very shy and unsociable, the other intending to marry and in need of support to free himself of the family without undue feelings of guilt vis-a-vis his father. Not all of the sons have been very lucky in finding a partner. I know that one of them has chosen an orphan and another a severely mentally disturbed girl. The emotional climate in their families leaves much to be desired and already the children are showing signs of maladaptations. I am afraid therefore that there is reason to believe that the impact of the premature death of the mother in family Geranium is going to have repercussions not only in the second, but also in the third generation, perhaps going on indefinitely.

This family history illustrates the interplay between nature and nurture very well. The tubercolosis of the mother spread to the father and one of

43

the children. Several of the children inherited her sebaceous skin, giving rise to endless infections and cysts and to recurring otitis externa. Perhaps it is note-worthy in this connection that the mother had a herpes zoster in 1949, as had the eldest daughter in 1950, the youngest in 1954 and the fifth son in 1961. I know that at least two of the children showed signs of the same inner ear deafness as the mother. Two sons had a prolapsed disc at an unusually young age (one aged 15 years old, operation being necessary, and another at 19) and I think it highly probable that the schizoid trait of the father has played a role in the development of the character of several of his children. But it is utterly impossible to draw a sharp dividing line between the inner (hereditary) influences and outer (environmental) circumstances in the medical life history of this family.

B.   Mrs. Hyacinth was a heavy but lively woman with reddish hair. The impression she gave was in marked contrast to her mother, who was slow and passive, talking with a low drawling voice and giving the impression of permanent exhaustion. I began to understand this difference better when I discovered that her mother had a Simmonds disease or pituitary cachexia due to a severe haemorrhage after the birth of her youngest child.

Mr. Hyacinth was an unskilled labourer in the building trade. He, too, was heavy and all their ten children were like this, several of them arriving in the world with difficulty, due to their big shoulders causing problems at delivery.

In addition to her ten children Mrs. Hyacinth also had had two miscarriages. In the spring of 1955, 18 months after her last delivery, she consulted me because she felt pain in her left breast. The skin there looked like the skin of an orange and I palpated a hard mass in the depth and a second mass in the region of her axilla. The clinical picture did not differ much from that of a mastitis she had after her ninth delivery, but she was not now breast feeding. I referred Mrs. Hyacinth to the surgeon who agreed to operate on her and found a medullary carcinoma as we had already feared. After the removal of her breast combined with clearance of the axilla, she had radiotherapy. I saw her in June to remove some stitches. She was complaining of nausea due to the irradiation and in the same month she started to complain of backpain. In July I sent Mrs. Hyacinth to the radiologist, who could not find anything abnormal, but the pains became worse and in August several collapsed vertebrae due to metastases were found. The haemoglobin fell in a very short time from 35 to 20%. The blood picture was that of aplastic anaemia and despite transfusions and further radiotherapy Mrs. Hyacinth died within a few weeks at the age of 41.

After her death the younger children were sent to relatives and friends, but they returned in a very short time, because they produced problems, none of them being toilet trained. This fits into the picture of this large sloppy family, as do the many skin infections and accidents (see chart 11a

44

and 11b, appendix 2), some of them being very serious, like fractures due to falls out of the window. A nun came to stay with the family for a few months, but afterwards they looked after themselves, although a sister of Mrs. Hyacinth kept some sort of supervision.

As can be seen from the charts, after a few years six of the children left the family, none of them because of marriage, which is an unusual event in a family like this. This can be interpreted as a demonstration of the effect of the loss of the functional axis of the mother in the family. Three boys went into the navy, similar to the family Geranium, where three boys went into a seminary.

With the girls the story was somewhat different. The eldest daughter, who had to carry the burden of the housekeeping for this large family, started in 1956 to complain of abdominal pains. She was admitted to hospital with suspected appendicitis, but this diagnosis could not be confirmed. She alleged she had her periods every fortnight but she proved to be an inaccurate and vague historian, and the gynaecologist could not find anything abnormal. She kept complaining about her abdomen, and later of several other symptoms, for which no physical cause could be detected. It became clear that the burden of the family was too heavy for her. In 1958 she had again to be admitted to hospital for an investigation of her severe abdominal pains; again nothing abnormal could be established. The next year she ran away from home and never returned.

The second daughter came to carry the burden now. As in family Geranium she was very strict with the other children (the neighbours told me), allowing them no freedom at all. But she managed to hold on, perhaps because she had a part time job outside the family. In 1961 she began to have nervous symptoms and in 1962 she also started to complain about her abdomen. She was married in 1963.

Before she left the house for a resident job with another family, the third daughter visited my surgery several times in 1961, with tummy aches, but nothing was found on examination. At the moment, in 1977, the youngest daughter is looking after the family. She complains only occasionally about headaches and seems to hold up well. She is on good terms with her father and her brothers. She is engaged and I see her regularly because she is using the pill. When I visit the house now, it strikes me that it is cleaner and more pleasant than it has ever been before.

But we (the social worker, the district nurse, the priest and I) have had a lot of worry about child number 8, Charles, who was five years old when his mother died. He had many accidents and when he was eleven he started to steal and to start fires. Charles was sent to a boarding school from which he returned in 1965. Nobody in the whole family is very clever, but his intelligence is definitely below normal. He has already been admitted to hospital four times for episodes of concussion and his EEG shows abnormalities. He does not like work and has great difficulties in finding his place in society.

When we look at the history of this family Hyacinth it is striking to see that, just as in the three previous families, there is a latent period of some years before the impact of the loss of one of the parents begins to manifest itself in the medical history. Then the threatening disintegration becomes apparent and nervous symptoms begin to appear. The family system tries to preserve its existence at the expense of the health of its individual members. The stories of the daughters give us a clear example of the family patterning of illness; they choose the same symptoms. The unusually high incidence of skin infections and accidents in all members of family Geranium and Hyacinth gives us new evidence of the importance of the family as a unit of illness.

C.   I first met Mrs. Iris (chart 12, appendix 2) in labour when I arrived in this practice March 1943. Luckily all went well, except for a perineal tear which I had to repair. She was a kindhearted and motherly, plump woman, with a pale chubby face and bulging heavy-spectacled eyes. Later I delivered six further babies and came to know Mrs. Iris very well. She was a daughter of a local farmer, but her husband came from a big city in the west of the country and was a motor mechanic. His brother had started a flourishing garage in the neighbouring town and had asked him to come and help. Afraid of being on call night and day if he lived close to the garage, Mr. Iris put an advertisement in the newspaper for lodgings elsewhere and so he came to live in our village with the parents of his future wife. He was seven years younger than she and possibly he was looking for a wife with a mother-image.

In 1943 Mr. Iris consulted me several times for recurrent sycosis barbae and in the autumn of that year he was deported to Germany. He managed to escape from the slave labour camp by exaggerating his hallux valgus. I referred him to an orthopaedic surgeon, but his operation was postponed until the war was over.

The first serious blow to his family came in 1951 when the seventh pregnancy of Mrs. Iris resulted in a precipitous labour, the child dying after some days due to cerebral haemorrhage. In the sixth month of her next pregnancy Mrs. Iris started to vomit and to feel unwell. Her urine was of a dark colour and appeared to contain bile pigments. In a short time she became jaundiced and severely ill. Labour started, and a premature girl was born who died after a few hours. The condition of Mrs. Iris deteriorated rapidly, despite admission to the hospital and she died the next day, with the clinical picture of acute yellow atrophy of the liver, at the age of 41. The etiology of this dramatic illness became apparent when within a fortnight of her death four of her children developed simple infectious hepatitis.

Six weeks after the death of his wife, Mr. Iris came to my surgery complaining of shortness of breath and palpitations. He looked pale and

46

his pulse-rate was 140. His haemoglobin was 50% and his stools contained blood. X-rays confirmed the presence of an active duodenal ulcer and I had to advise him to rest in bed. He had a housekeeper who looked after his children. She came from a convent in France, a nervous and tense young woman, who tried to do her best. She brought with her a prescription for a sedative from the psychotherapist, who evidently had advised her to leave the convent. Mr. Iris told me later, that in the cold winter nights, she came down to sleep in his bed, being completely ignorant in sexual effairs. Notwithstading initial difficulties in intercourse, she soon became pregnant, which pregnancy ended in a spontaneous abortion. Her uterus was very small with a long pointed cervix.

They started to have qualms of conscience, and she presented Mr. Iris with the choice either to marry her or to let her go. He chose the first solution, though he did not love her at that time. Although they had a difficult life together in the beginning, afterwards he came to love her, as he told me later. She was not able to cope with the children of Mr. Iris' first marriage, but things went better after she had children of her own.

They got into serious financial difficulties. Mr. Iris had started a business in bicycles and motorcycles which prospered, but after his first wife's death he lost interest and sold his property in order to emigrate to Australia. Unfortunately at the time of the medical examination he happened to have a transient bronchitis and was rejected. He found a job driving, mostly away from home, but worried about how things were going with the family. On his returns he found the two things he disliked most of all, quarrels and disorder. Mr. Iris soon had his second bleeding and had an operation for his peptic ulcer. After this he started as a truckdriver, and had to carry heavy loads, resulting in a prolapsed disc, which forced him to a third period of bedrest. He then started as a bus driver, compelled to keep to the clock and feeling frustrated in the traffic, giving rise to new stomach aches. He then resumed his work as a mechanic, became an expert in diesel motors which he enjoyed and was held in high esteem by his employer. He had a very good income, supplemented by buying and selling second-hand cars, but his wife was unable to budget, and they were always short of money. Mr. Iris felt ashamed that his brothers and sisters had attained a higher social status, and he constantly dreamt of being able to start a garage of his own with his sons. When he finally succeeded in this, it was as a manager away from my practice, and so this family left my care after I had witnessed it through its most difficult period.

The first four families which I described, having lost a parent, tried to continue to function as they had before, for as long as possible, illustrating the concept of the family as a homeostatic system. In this fifth family it was clear to each member from the beginning, that its structure had to change. There was a lot of resistance against this from the elder children, and many tensions between them and the new mother, who had her own children in great pain and anxiety, due to her ambivalence and insecurity. But then an escape-mechanism in family dynamics came into action; a scapegoat. The fourth child, John, had difficulties at school with arithmetic and he behaved peculiarly at school and home. In 1956 he was blamed by the family as the cause of most of its problems, and without realizing what was going on exactly, I referred him to a child guidance clinic.

The child psychiatrist wrote me a letter in return, stating that John was of normal intelligence, but had a specific weakness in maths. He appeared neurotic, the family situation being very unsuitable for this sensitive and nervous boy. A special school was advised, and a social caseworker would try to ease the attitude of his step-mother.

Three years later, John's condition did not appear to have improved, and a second opinion was deemed to be necessary. I had a long interview with Mrs. Iris, in which she confided all her problems. She could not get along with her step-children and she felt very guilty about this, especially about John. She confessed to me that she realized that his development was her fault. Not all the money of the world would permit her to confess this to the social caseworker by whom she felt humiliated. She felt very lonely and isolated in this village, unable to relate with other women. She had serious financial and sexual problems, being frightened of further pregnancies and told me she contemplated suicide. I was deeply impressed by her story and when I got home I did what I should have done long ago, I consulted my records and found that I had noted as long ago as 1950, when his own mother was still in full health, that John was a peculiar boy. His nursery teacher told me his only answer to all questions was "yes". He had whooping cough when he was very young, and a serious attack of measles at the age of two.

This information enabled me to reduce Mrs. Iris's feelings of guilt in subsequent long interviews, which improved our relationship. John did much better when he got his first job, and even learned to count when he started to earn and spend his own money, and this improved the internal relationship in the Iris's family. When they left the practice in 1961 I reviewed their records with benefit at that time, tracing not only family epidemics of trichophyton, otitis media, bronchitis, pneumonia, mumps. measles, whooping cough, chickenpox, pyodermia, strophulus, conjunctivitis, rubella and infectious hepatitis, but especially the dynamic interactions of this family.

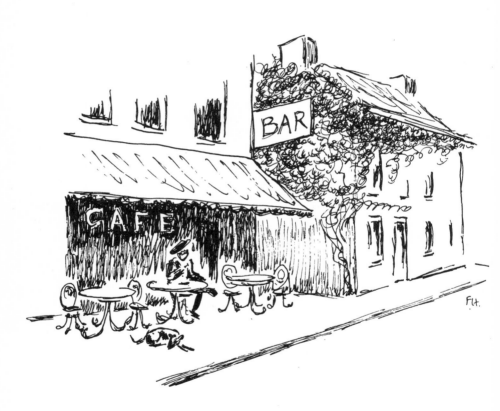

VII. Family-patterning in Illness

A.   Mrs. Jasmin lived with her only son on whom she relied heavily (see chart 13, appendix 2). Her husband had died when he was 58, her three daughters were married. She and her son ran an inn and a paint shop. Mrs. Jasmin needed a pessary for her vaginal prolapse and required a visit several times a year to change it as she could not come to me due to her arthritis.

In 1949 she developed all kinds of nervous symptoms including aerophagy and sleeplessness, but she localized these in her abdomen. Except for a single attack of cystitis in 1951, I could never find anything wrong in her abdomen. Neither could the specialist in internal medicine whom she consulted. At first I did not understand what was making her ill, but in 1953 it became clear that she was worrying about her son. She wanted him to marry, now that she was getting old. He promised to do so but he never did. I could have given this chapter the title of "the man who did not dare to marry".

He was engaged to a girl who had lost her parents when she was 18 and who then looked after her old uncle and aunt. When they died in 1954, she did not know where to go so she came to live in the house of Mrs. Jasmin and helped in the pub. Mr. Jasmin promised he would marry her soon. At first Mrs. Jasmin was pleased with this, as she believed that her son now really was about to marry, but soon serious tensions began to rise between her and her son, and also between her and her future daughter-in-law. Mrs. Jasmin's endless whining complaints about her abdomen and other symptoms became unbearable.

In December 1955 she fled to her daughter who lived in the city, hoping with this manoeuvre to trap her son in two respects: he was now living alone in the house with his fiancée and the social pressure of the village would force him to get married. The license of the pub was in her name and this gave her a mighty second weapon. She hoped to be able to return in triumph soon, but Mr. Jasmin did not weaken. In fact they never met again. The son did not go to see her and as far as I know they never even wrote to each other. As I continued to look after her in the city, they tried to bargain via me. She gave in regarding the license when the son earnestly promised to marry but he was unable to keep this promise. They longed for each other and they always eagerly asked me how the other was doing, but they were unable to bridge the gap between them. The tragedy was, that in my opinion, the mother herself unconsciously was the cause which prevented her son from ever marrying.

In the meantime pressure rose in the family of her daughter. The complaints of Mrs. Jasmin upset the atmosphere so that the children left home. They were not patients of mine, but they started to frequent their general practitioner and at the weekends the husband often came to my door, in tears of misery. In 1957 they refused to have her with them any longer and they sent her to an old people's home in another town where she died two years later.

Mr. Jasmin was trapped indeed. He started to develop severe asthmatic attacks which incapacitated him in a few years by a supervening emphysema. It is true that his first asthmatic attack had happened in 1948, before he was trapped socially, and he told me that his mother's father and his father's mother both had been asthmatic. But there is no doubt that his attacks occurred more frequently as his frustration increased, and that his condition deteriorated with unusual rapidity. He had to be admitted many times to a chest-hospital, often in a critical state, short of breath, cyanotic and almost unconscious. Because he would not consent to being admitted unless he was very near death, I feared several times he would not reach the hospital alive. The strange thing is that he also, like his mother, localized his complaints in his abdomen. He never spoke about his lungs or his asthma but always of his stomach as the cause of his distress.

Mr. Jasmin stopped painting and he stopped playing the organ in the church, though he still could have done this very well physically, and he stopped going outdoors, because he did not dare to come in contact with his neighbours and fellow-villagers any longer. He did not come into his own bar and resigned himself to bed more and more, while he was most unco-operative in his medical treatment. I arranged for a social worker to help him solve his problems. I was afraid that his fiancée was going to have to pay the penalty if he were to die, for even though she had now run the inn for years, his relatives were eager to throw her out of his house and keep the license to themselves. The social worker had many interviews with both of them and they agreed hesitantly to marry. He was too embarrassed to go to the town hall, being ashamed that he was ill and getting old, but the social worker succeeded in persuading the authorities to come to their house for the ceremony. At the final date, Mr. Jasmin found some excuse to postpone the ceremony for a few days; in the meantime he had to be admitted to hospital again where he suddenly died with the signs and symptoms of a pneumonia.

Luckily things had been arranged in time with the lawyer. Mr. Jasmin's fiancée inherited his house and she is now, in 1977, still running the bar. She has a definite social function in this community, giving support to other lonely and socially handicapped people. Like the old mother she is also fat now and crippled by arthritis. I should mention that she too had abdominal troubles. Soon after she came into this family her gallstone problems started and she had an operation for these. I do not think this to be a mere coincidence, as it is known that there are definite correlations between gallstone-trouble and emotional tension. Recently she had to be operated upon for the second time, a stone in the bile duct giving rise to intermittent obstruction. Strangely enough it took considerable effort to convince the specialist of this diagnosis, as he was thinking of some kind of hepatitis, but this was very unlikely at her age in the view of most general practitioners. I even had to send her to a second radiologist who localized the stone by tomography.

One of the daughters of Mrs. Jasmin stayed in my practive after her marriage. When we look at the diagram of her family (Family Kingcup, chart 14, appendix 2) it is at once clear that she also was a high-user of the doctor's services. This pattern is constant over the years, with the exception of the war, when it was the general experience of all doctors in Holland that medical demands diminished considerably whilst the stresses of life increased.

Analysing the medical episodes of her life history, we find the usual disorders connected with her sexual-reproductive functions such as recurrent urinary infections, abortion, post partum haemorrhage, anaemia, varicose veins and ulcers etc. But it also transpires that, like her mother, she complained again and again about her abdomen. She, too, became abnormally fat and was constantly wondering what might be wrong in her enormous belly. We consulted a medical specialist several times, who sent back numerous reports. In his first letter he stressed an elevated sedimentation rate and mentioned the possibility of cholecystitis. In his second letter he considered gallstones, without being able to demonstrate them. In his third letter he mentioned she might have chronic appendicitis and in his fourth letter the remote chance of allergy. It was in his fifth letter, at last, that he confessed being unable to find anything wrong in his field, and he suggested a gynaecologist should see her, which resulted in the finding of a physiological cervical erosion.

On the patient's request she was later sent to another medical specialist, and finally to a psychiatrist, but none of them could offer any real help. On the contrary, they all led us astray, doing endless investigations, without finding the real cause of her troubles. This story is a good illustration I think, of the little help a general practitioner can expect from specialists in the management of this type of problem.

More relevant to her management was my discovery in '55-'56 that she worried about the arguments in her mother's family, and later about her husband's tendency to drink excessively. I could understand his failure for several reasons. His occupation in the building trade exposed him to parties and social drinking and his wife's endless complaining drove him frantic over the weekends, even leading him to phone me in desperation. Alcoholism is notoriously difficult to treat, but in his case nature came to help us, as his abuse of alcohol precipitated bouts of paroxysmal tachycardia, which forced him to stop drinking. The many and often serious accidents in this family (see chart 14a, appendix 2) perhaps may have some relation to his alcoholism, a fact I have often observed in families with an alcoholic father.

Later the mother started to worry about her children as they were going to marry. Chart 14b (appendix 2) gives us a picture of the incidence of nervous troubles in this family, giving rise to requests for medical care. Everyone who studies this figure will see clearly that this mother succeeded in transmitting her own and her mother's symptoms to each of her children. Several of them have developed overt neurotic behaviour such as frank agorophobia. Only one of them (child no. 4) stayed my patient after her marriage. As happens so often she succeeded in finding a partner of almost identical personality and proneness to neurosis. Both husband and wife are constantly in need of help for all kinds of nervous symptoms. There have been serious coital difficulties, needing behaviour therapy by a psychologist, and both lost one job after the other, due to problems of adaptation.

The eldest daughter, child no. 3, who came back home in 1975 has taken to drinking and has been divorced.

No one in this family developed their uncle's asthma, although the mother has had symptoms of hay fever and eczema. But I think the incidence of lower respiratory tract disorders (chart 14c appendix 2) is interesting, because it shows the unusual frequency of bronchitis during 1947-1948, when they lived in a small wooden shed with overcrowding and frequent temperature changes. Again this demonstrates the interplay between internal and external factors in producing disease in families.

B.   I do not know what Mr. Lavender's health was before or during the war, because I only came to know him in 1947 when he returned from imprisonment for political offences, having been a collaborator with the Nazi's during the occupation. I recall him as a submissive and gloomy man, but it may be that my early memory is coloured by his final history and by the Parkinson's disease he also had in the end. It is quite certain that he was often ill after returning as proved by a figure I made in 1962 (see chart 15, appendix 2) for a lecture. His symptoms were always very vague and, as can be seen, I referred him several times to specialists, who usually said they could not find much either, and thought him fit for work. In 1948 he probably had a duodenal ulcer and in 1957 he had an operation for his prostate gland, but these somatic findings could not explain his usual host of symptoms and his preference to stay in bed. He stopped becoming ill in 1959, probably because he had his pension then and did not have to work any longer.

His wife was also often ill, but not exceptionally for a woman of that age, although the number of referrals (8 in the chart) was higher than my average. As can be anticipated, many of her episodes of illness were related to sexual-reproductive problems. She had a prolapse, which disappeared later spontaneously during her menopause, and she suffered from varicose veins with ulcers. She always seemed to have recurring urinary infections, for which I referred her to a medical specialist, then a surgeon and later again to an urologist, who considered the cause to be urethritis and vaginitis due to her habit of vaginal douching with water. He advised instead regular vulval cleansing with oil after micturition and this simple advice brought an end to her urinary infections. She suffered recurrent abdominal symptoms, perhaps due to colonic diverticulosis that had been demonstrated, and also she had rosacea.

When we look at the diagram for nervous symptoms (chart 15, appendix 2) it is clear that these started after her husband returned in 1947. Five of her children had already left home, and as we see three of the others followed in the period of observation. All children were frequently ill, having all kinds of nervous symptoms, expressed in physical complaints such as tiredness, headaches, dizziness, pain over the heart with palpitations, with pain in the back being a particular favourite of this family. All these symptoms and the many minor accidents and even flu of no severity had one thing in common: in their opinion it rendered them always definitely unfit for work. When we look at the nervous symptoms in the diagram it appears that they increase, especially in the girls, when they grew up and were about to leave the family.

The medical history of the youngest member of this family, the boy born in 1936, illustrates the interaction more fully. In 1950 he told me that he was constantly passing urine, without being aware of this and I noted that he was continually blinking nervously. In 1953 he complained of pain between his shoulderblades, of headaches and vomiting, later of constipation and pain in his sides, in 1954 pain in the back and the next year loss of appetite and insomnia. Two years later it was headaches, pain in the throat, nervous coughing, tiredness and listlessness, in 1957 tinnitus, vague complaints about his eyes with headaches and at the end of that year during military service he often stayed on at home after weekend leave alleging headaches, stomach aches or pains in the chest. This boy remained my patient after his marriage, as did three of his brothers. He had to marry a 17 year old dull girl (related to another high-users family) because she was pregnant. The number of times this new young family sent for me is countless, usually for the same symptoms. It is perhaps significant to mention that this young man, already in his early thirties, was declared officially unfit for any work for the rest of his life, due to functional low backpains and now receives an invalidity-pension, although I see him regularly digging in his garden.

The situation with his brothers in this practice is not much better. In order to document the pattern of illness-behaviour in this family, I investigated in depth the family medical history of the eldest son, who married in 1943, before his father went to prison (chart 16, appendix 2).

A whole book could be filled with the medical history of this junior Mr. Lavender. He is an intelligent man with a pleasing appearance, well behaved, but his host of constantly recurring symptoms makes it onerous having to be his general practitioner during these years.

First he had gastric complaints, and it is true that twice he could have had a duodenal ulcer like his father, but later backache became predominant, and later still all kinds of cardiovascular symptoms. He had lots of complaints about his head and as well a whole series of accidents. One look at chart 16 will suffice to demonstrate how frequently he was ill. Perhaps this man has been off sick for more time than he has worked. It can be seen that I referred many, many times to specialists, with the exception of the last few years, when I learnt to my (and his) cost that specialists' advice is seldom helpful to this type of patient, and often even harmful. A neurologist for instance admitted him to hospital to assess a head injury that never really occurred, making it almost impossible for me to rehabilitate him afterwards. In the same year an orthopaedic surgeon to whom he went for the pain in his back, wrote first that he could not find anything significant, but three weeks later he advised the patient to go to bed for a month, advising me to mobilize him gradually after this. An E.N.T. surgeon, to whom I referred him with the question whether perhaps sinusitis could explain his headaches, thought this unlikely, but added in parenthesis that this "neuralgia" could be due to previous sinusitis.

It must be said that several of these many referrals to specialists were initiated during my holidays by locums, and several others by public health doctors who wanted to be sure whether this patient was fit for work or not. Nevertheless it can be stated that much iatrogenic damage resulted from referring somatic complaints to appropriate specialists. Nor with the seven psychiatrists were my experiences much better on the occasions when Mr. Lavender jr was seen by them. From the psychotherapist of 1946 I never received a reply. His colleague in 1950 wrote about a compensation neurosis and made some very good remarks about how this patient frustrated him. Never having had the opportunity of qualifying as a physiotherapist Mr. Lavender jr. was envious of doctors. I knew that he used to treat other patients as a quack and I noticed that he evidently tried to imitate me by wearing my kind of beret, owning the same breed of dog, letting his house become overgrown by the same kind of creeper and even being converted to his doctor's religion. The psychiatrist told him to ignore his pains, and to aim at being a normal person, offering to help him with this, but I am afraid that this advice did not much interest our patient. In 1952 a psychiatrist wrote about neuropathy, a psychotherapist about neurasthenia and a third neuropsychiatrist about a prolapsed disc, recommending admission to hospital. In 1953 a psychiatrist diagnosed Mr. Lavender jr. as having "hysterical neuropathy, or even simulating" and in 1961 yet another psychiatrist was sure we were dealing with severe depression, possibly endogenous, worsened by a "stress", this being that his wife overspent, causing financial problems. In reality I knew that this wife was earning money by working while our patient stayed at home, the psychiatrist having stated that he was unfit to work for six months. So psychiatrists appeared to be of as little practical value as the specialists in organic disease.

In my opinion the social worker has done far better in helping this man and his family. Several times she improved things considerably when the outlook seemed hopeless.

I had several long evening interviews with this patient. He told me about his youth, having been beaten and abused by his father who hated him. In early life he was brought up by grandparents, because his parents were constantly quarreling about him. He used to say that his bad youth was the origin of all his troubles and it is almost tragic to observe that in spite of his childhood this patient copied his father's behaviour later in his marriage, possibly due to some compulsive repetition. He welcomed punishment both physical and mental, asking for severe treatment.

He married a small, pale but fine woman who until the very end seemed to have believed completely he was a sick man. He distressed her, particularly in the last ten years or so, by continually threatening suicide to end his suffering. He often slept with a knife under his pillow and she caught him several times in the barn toying with a rope, pretending to hang himself. All this was done to emphasize to her that she had to comply or risk losing him suddenly. She was seriously impressed by all his symptoms, so endured much without ever uttering a single complaint to me. But, as chart 16 shows in 1961 she too began to get nervous symptoms which slowly worsened over the following years. In the last few years she even began to thwart her husband, giving rise to conflicts. When in 1973 he went so far as to take a young female divorced "patient" of his, with small children of whom he was going to be the foster-father, into his house, she refused to submit any more, fled to a married daughter and shortly afterwards obtained a divorce.

It can be seen from the same diagram that the two eldest daughters started to have nervous symptoms when they were twelve years old. It is significant that at a young age both of them started to complain about backaches, which is very unusual in children.

This three generation history well illustrates the importance of family-patterning of disease, a mechanism which must be well known to every experienced family doctor. Father transmitted it in this family, in contrast to the first family of this chapter, when it was transmitted by mother.

There is one final intriguing question: why has the youngest daughter escaped this fate? I have often observed in similar families, where mental illness is transmitted from one generation to the next, that some children escape this, and several examples of this phenomenon are found in the family histories related and charted in this book. The outcome does not seem to be predestined. What is the reason? Are these children born immune or do they become immune? It would be very worthwhile to investigate in which respect these children differ from their unhappy brothers and sisters, as this could point to ways of breaking the vicious link being transmitted from generation to generation.

VIII. Problem Families

A.   Every general practitioner has problem patients, making him sigh inwardly when he sees them entering his consulting room. Julie Marguerite was such a patient. She was born in 1935 (chart 17, appendix 2) and she was eight years old when I came to this practice. In the first years nothing peculiar struck me. She had the normal diseases of her age. In 1944 I referred her to an E.N.T. surgeon for tonsillectomy for her recurrent tonsillitis. In 1947 she started to come for pains in her legs for which I could find no cause. The next year I referred her to the E.N.T. surgeon again, because she kept complaining of her throat. I should never have done this because after her second operation the symptoms only worsened. In 1949 she had a metatarsal fracture but in 1950 her complaints were of her tumm and shortness of breath, both symptoms being typically nervous in nature. I saw she was a fat and clumsy girl. Next year she complained of all manner of pains in her legs and she had red marks on her skin suggestive of scratching, with made me think of an artefact. The dermatologist, to whom I referred her, did not agree as he found erythrocyanosis, but he could not explain her severe pains. He prescribed large doses of vitamin D2 but I found that the only way to heal her leg ulcers was by occlusive bandaging in order to prevent her from scratching. Later she produced the red marks on her face, so possibly my original diagnosis was correct. In 1952 I referred her back to the E.N.T. specialist because she persistently complained of aches in her ears and throat for which he did a third tonsillectomy. In retrospect I realize I may have subconsciously used those referrals as a means of punishing her. In August I referred her to an orthopaedic surgeon for the pains in her legs. He, of course, found flat feet and diagnosed general muscular irritability from her feet to her long spinal muscles. His first letter stated that the complaints were definitely of postural origin and I can still feel some of his irritation while I read this opinion as I had specifically mentioned that I suspected psychological causes. He admitted her to hospital for a thorough course of physical therapy, but after some time he discharged her rather abruptly, stating in his final report that ultimately he had come to the conclusion that the cause of her troubles must be psychogenic.

He must have written similarly to the doctor who examined her for a job application in 1954, and to whom she alleged that she had been treated by the orthopaedic surgeon for a dislocated hip. As a result she was rejected. She kept returning to my surgery more and more often with every sort of complaint and manifestation. It is interesting to re-read my notes and find that during each of my holidays, she was one of the first to try out my locum. She would have symptoms for all variety of ailments and although she often hinted at appendicitis, it took her 3 years to find a locum who did not trust his own opinion and passed her, and the diagnosis, on to a surgeon. Of course the surgeon could find no signs of an appendicitis or nephrolithiasis, but once having gained access to him, she kept returning and, as happens so often, in self defence he finally opened her abdomen and found, needless to say, nothing wrong. My experience is that almost every surgeon will operate eventually if the patient turns up sufficiently often. Perhaps it is more dangerous for a patient to consult an irascible surgeon than an irritated family doctor, though the danger of the family doctor missing serious organic disease by this preoccupation is not to be underestimated. Julie gave her surgeon various opportunities to operate on her again but he declined.

September the ninth 1960 she came, stating that she had not had a bowel movement for a fortnight. More significant it appeared on questioning that her period was a week overdue, a few days later the urine pregnancy test returned positive. Then she told me that she had been attacked and raped by two unknown men, but confessed afterwards that this was not true, the truth being that she had gone to a party, had drunk too much, and had had intercourse with several of her loose boyfriends.

It is usual and customary to attach the appropriate diagnostic label to this sort of medical history: a classic example of hysteria. But this does not help us in treating the patient. It is much more useful to ask oneself why this kind of behaviour happened. If we do this, it emerges that Julie was the daughter of a couple living in marital disharmony and conflicts. Her father was originally a broker, the son of a well-to-do but very aggressive man. Her mother came from a fine, intellectual family, several of them occupying high church positions, of which she was very proud. I am afraid that she always felt slightly superior to her husband, and this increased when he started drinking. After quarreling with his father, he lost his money by foolish business transactions, ran into debt, went bankrupt and had to accept inferior jobs. He failed time and again, ran up further debts, escaped into alcohol and finally indulged in fraud. His medical history tells of fractures and other accidents, low back pains and attempts to stop drinking.

In the beginning, his wife rescued him several times by paying his debts with her money, and when her money was gone she borrowed from relatives. Following the advice of her clerical family, she soon ceased this financial help. The marriage ended in divorce in 1960. Her medical history consisted of recurrent episodes of tonsillitis and a tonsillectomy, of muscular and other vague rheumatic symptoms, with referrals to an orthopaedic surgeon and several other specialists and culminated in all sorts of nervous symptoms.

Julie disliked her mother but was fond of her father and felt deserted when he left the family. Shortly thereafter she became pregnant, perhaps seeking compensation for her loneliness and at the same time defying her mother. She never gave me the impression of being too unhappy with·her pregnancy. Her mother made a desperate effort to hide the truth by moving. Julie had her baby in hospital, kept it and was glad. Afterwards she married and had twins. At first all seems to have gone well in her marriage, but later I heard she too was divorced.

Her elder sister seems to have made a better marriage, although there have been rumours of problems. My notes show that she developed all kinds of functional complaints, headaches, backpains, stomach aches, tiredness and so on, when she was about 18 years old. She was referred to a medical specialist who excluded organic disease. She seemed contrary to her sister, Julie, close to her mother.

The eldest brother of Julie was of limited physical and intellectual capacities. He was fat (as insecure boys often are) and frequently came to me with doubtful or very insignificant disorders, which gave him an excuse to stay away from his work and his military service. Socially he became more or less a failure. He never married and sought protection in a humle sheltered administrative job with a safe pension.

The tragedy of this family culminated in the fate of the youngest son, Paul, a nice boy. In his youth he had the usual children's diseases and several small accidents. In the autumn of 1949, when he was 12 years old, he went to a seminary to become a priest, and I have no doubt that his respect and adoration of his mother's brothers was a powerful factor in his choice. But he soon came back, being constantly ill at the seminary. I could find no cause for his illness. I was told that his temperature was always raised, but the E.S.R. was normal, as were all agglutinations and other tests. He said that he longed to return when fit, and I referred him to a medical specialist, an ophthalmologist and a neurologist respectively, as he kept complaining of unbearable headaches. He stayed in bed for months, but his temperature and symptoms disappeared suddenly when it was decided that he should not return to the seminary. I suspect that he was constantly trying to fall in with his mother's deepest wishes without really being able to fulfil them. So instead of the seminary, he went to navigation school and in 1957 he went to sea. He wrote kind letters to his mother from ports all over the world and sent her all his earnings. I saw Paul again on November the fifteenth 1960 at 13.00 hours, after entering his locked room in the attic. He was in a deep coma with all reflexes absent, including the corneal reflex and the light reflex of the pupil. He had come home at 12 o'clock the night before, after a quarrel with his fiancée and it appeared that he had taken an enormous dose of sleeping tablets. I sent him to hospital and he was rescued from death's door, staying in hospital for several weeks. The psychiatrist reported at his discharge that he had a reactive depression due to the breaking off of the engagement by his fiancée.

This engagement was re-established officially on the first of January 1961, but, as I heard afterwards, broken again by the girl four days later. On the fifth day of the year he was found dead in a hotel in Amsterdam, where he had taken a room under the name of a Swedish sailor. He had been heard snoring, but nobody paid any attention to this until it was too late.

I went to Paul's mother to talk with her. She told me that he had been looking forward to his long leave, but when he came home he soon became depressed and cried constantly. This was put down to his finding a broken home and a pregnant sister. His mother was full of guilt over his death and the pregnancy of her daughter. She believed these to be a punishment for her going through with the divorce, although she and her relatives realized that this was the best solution. Most of all she was concerned about the salvation of her son's soul.

I had a talk later with one of her brothers who was a priest and from him I learned that his sister had been bodily tortured by her husband, a secret sadist, from the beginning of her marriage. The husband could not stand his son who resembled him, and always beat him until Paul grew stronger than he was. Paul twice saw his married sister who told me he talked about his fear of becoming like his father. His girlfriend was of a considerably lower social level and they had been having intercourse over a long period of time. The psychiatrist to whom I went afterwards with my feelings of guilt, asking him if it would not have been better to have kept this boy somewhat longer in hospital, told me then that indeed he knew Paul had been a sadist: he could not come to a sexual climax unless he was aggressive and hurt his girl, this being the reason she broke the engagement. Paul realized that he had inherited this tendency from his father and according to the psychiatrist he did not want to give up this trait. The psychiatrist spoke of him as of a deeply disturbed psychopathic personality with a very bad prognosis.

I went home and wondered how it was possible that all this had happened before my eyes, thinking that as their family doctor I knew these people very well, while in reality I had not understood what was going on under my nose. I had been their general practitioner true enough, but I had not been their family doctor. Instead of referring them to various specialists (as a way of defence) I should have recognized the family dynamics underlying their behaviour and should have tried to help them with these.

B.   Mrs. Mary Narcissus has been my patient since her marriage in 1952 (chart 18, appendix 2). I usually address her as Mary because she once asked me to do so, and so I know that she likes this. It is strange to realize that one addresses some people with their Christian name and others with "Mr", "Mrs" or "Miss", still after a long time in the same practice. When students come to sit in with me, they usually ask after the first day or two why this is so, and it is sometimes difficult to explain exactly on which grounds one makes the distinction.

Mary was several months pregnant when she married, and later I understood that this had been necessary in order to get the consent of her mother. She lost her father due to an acute throat disease on her fourteenth birthday and her mother was left with 12 children.

Her first baby was born within four months of her marriage and was named after herself, as a first daughter. The delivery took place in the emergency housing they had been able to get, which was one of a row of 16 erected hastily after the war. At first these very simple dwellings had been occupied by those villagers whose houses had been destroyed during the war, but they moved out as their houses were rebuilt and newcomers to the village took their place. With the decreasing shortage of housing some process of social sedimentation was taking place: the row of emergency dwellings developed gradually into a kind of slum, a phenomenon not known previously in our village. This in turn caused the social and mental morale of the inhabitants to fall. I saw several of the families which came to live there get into a vicious circle of lowered standards and I fear that this was the case with Mary's family.

Her second child was a boy, and so was called after his father. In her third pregnancy things started to go wrong: she had intermittent vaginal blood loss and labour started far too early. A premature child of 1000 gram was born and admitted to hospital, where it died in its first day. At that time it was already evident that Mary's husband was drinking heavily. He was a very nice and handsome boy with black hair and tanned skin, whom I had known since 1943, as his parents belonged to my practice. His father was a professional soldier and his education had been very disciplined.

The son was an adventurer who went to fight in Korea as a volunteer three times. He had hoped to be accepted as a professional soldier after this (like two of his brothers), but his request was rejected. He was very disappointed by this and felt unhappy for years looking back upon his military time with nostalgia. It was in Korea that he had learned to drink, having been almost forced to it as he told me. I had a long interview with him. He could not hold on to his various jobs, being unhappy, and left one after the other. He would then go on a drinking spree, not daring to go home and tell his wife. I wanted to refer him to a clinic for alcoholism to see if they could cure him of his habit, but he preferred to do it independently. He did not succeed in this and serious problems started to arise in his home and marriage. I had a second long interview with him. He developed a new interest and said that he wanted to go to sea. When he did so, he was very happy with the life, but he still could not refrain from drinking. So the couple decided in 1956 to join ship as a family, Mary hoping that this would reduce his drinking. They stayed away for nearly two years, while Mary returned once during that time to inform me she was going to get a divorce. Instead of this, she was pregnant again when the family came home in the beginning of 1958. Her second daughter was born after a very protracted and tiring labour, perhaps due to her ambivalence in having this child. In her lying-in period she had bronchial asthma, but neither the chest physician nor I could explain her subsequent lengthy fever, and I wrote in my notes that I thought this to be of nervous origin. In 1959 she had an abortion, which necessitated curettage, but it was in 1960 that she started to come with serious complaints such as fear of heartdisease, sudden death, of cancer, worries which continued the next few years, day and night.

The family situation deteriorated rapidly, with the usual ups and downs of alcoholism. Furniture was destroyed in rows, and twice all possessions were sold to pay off debts, the family having to sleep on old newspapers on the floor. But still the debts kept rising. Mary's husband was very clever and a smooth talker and could even borrow money from the alcoholic clinic official, pretending to need this in order to catch his ship, but of course going straight to the pub. He got a duodenal ulcer (like his father) which bled several times, but he was unable to rest in bed and his periods of abstinence became shorter. He could do with remarkably little rest, in fact he was unable to stay in bed for more than a few hours. I have often noted that alcoholics have sleep disturbances which leads me to believe that in some way their sleep-centre is disturbed. I had several long interviews with him again, whilst the social worker, the district nurse, the priest and I often conferred about Mary's ambivalence. She often talked to me about the possibility of divorce, but at the same time she asked the priest to regularize her marriage, as her husband was not a Roman Catholic, and to baptize her youngest child. Meanwhile she told the social worker about her troubles with her children and her fears that her son was going to develop his father's character, while at the same time she contemplated having yet another child because her husband wished this. It became clear that she was seriously entrapped in her life situation, unable to choose which way to turn. All of us pitied her as we watched her going round and round in an endless circle. Then I decided to attempt a series of long interviews with her, using Roger's technique of non-directive counseling, hoping to help her to reach a decision. With her consent I recorded these interviews on tape and they were analyzed in my Balintgroup afterwards with the assistance of a social psychiatrist. The decision she eventually made was to get a divorce although not before she had a fourth child. She put the onus on her husband to leave her, which he did, after which she at last got a new house. She managed to keep him out when he came back, drunk and hammering on her door with loud demands to be let in. I did not see him again as he went to live in Belgium with his second wife by whom he had a child. Mary told me he was lucky there, for he won the first prize in the national lottery and bought a big public house with his fortune. But still he kept drinking which led to two more operations for his peptic ulcer, till after the second operation he died from a pulmonary embolism in 1970 at the early age of 43.

Mary named her youngest son after me, which I found embarrassing. I gleaned from the long interviews that she had fallen in love with someone of a higher social level, who did not know this, and even adding later that this had happened because she told him all her troubles. She never got rid of her anxiety, as can be seen from the diagram, and until recently always presented her tension in somatic disguise. Almost 400 contacts are recorded between us. Orthodox medicine was of no use to her, neither did the many interviews which she had with the social worker lead to real progress. She kept complaining in the same way over these 12 years of difficulties with one child after the other and yet she never asked how far this could be due to herself.

She treated her children as adults ("parentiying"), leaning heavily upon them, and failed to give them a mother's warmth and security, so it is little wonder that they started to have nervous symptoms at an earlier age than usual, as can be seen in the chart. They also began to show behaviour-problems and there appeared to be no alternative to sending her eldest son to a boarding school for many years, for she kept recognizing her husband in this nice boy who did well when he was away from home and her. It was almost inevitable that the youngest son should take away small sums of money from his mother when he was eight years old and when Mary discovered this, she beat him nearly half dead in her panic. Family-patterning of illness was also revealed in the phenomenon that the three eldest children mimicked their mother's symptoms, coming to my surgery with pains over the heart, breathlessness and other anxiety symptoms. Even with their physical health it is interesting to note that three children had the same troubles, recurrent bronchitis and otitis media as did their mother, while the eldest daughter had serious infantile eczema. Both boys had febrile convulsions then too.

Mary went to work again after her divorce, having already done so before to solve her husband's debts and is now enjoying being a part-time help in the homes of elderly people. I hear from my old patients that she is highly appreciated. We got her to do this during her worst phase by persuading her to care for an old and lonely, incapacitated lady who had no one else to look after her. Mary made herself indispensable to this lady, did her shopping and purchased what seemed to me to be large quantities of cognac, a practice which proved most difficult to halt. It fascinated me to hear recently from the minister in our primary health care team (Mary has sought support from all denominations) that Mary phones him frequently in the evening and even in the middle of the night, quite evidently drunk; she now has alcohol problems herself and is trying to lean heavily on the minister, making me wonder in retrospect about the roots of her husband's drinking problems. Looking back on the story of this problem family, one thing is very clear to me: I made serious mistakes, as we all did. It was the classical error of having eyes only (or predominantly) for the poor, pitiful wife of the alcoholic. We should never have allowed her to become and to stay so dependent on us. We should not have focussed on her (or even on him) but on the relationship between them. We should have refrained from the many interviews with Mary, whereby we put her husband aside and isolated him still further. Their problems required combined or family therapy. It may be true that it is easy to draw conclusions after the event and that the development of family therapy is a recent advance, but I have written this story down hoping that it may convey a lesson to those of my readers who may meet the same pitfall to-morrow.

C.   It is difficult to give an accurate description of Mrs. Orchid, although I have known her for some 25 years and have met her often in all circumstances. There is something peculiar about her, she definitely is not very clever and sometimes I even think that she is backward, but at other times her remarks are very sensible. She is somewhat childish, looking upon you with wide, innocent, blue eyes and she is not unsympathetic. Life has been unkind to her. She married a singularly primitive cattle-dealer descended from a strange family, having something gipsy-like about them, and she had to live with her mother-in-law, a sharp, shrewd and exacting old lady, who grew up in a public house and was miserly with her money. In the first years Mrs. Orchid not only had to look after an unmarried brother of her husband, but also had to live next door to a married brother of his, with whom endless quarrels went on, though her husband shared the firm with him. So she lived in the middle of constant family feuds.

When we have a look at the diagram of this family (chart 19, appendix 2) we see that they have not sought much medical advice, which surprises me a little. But we must realize that I did not record the many contacts with the demanding grandmother, and the very many telephone calls by neighbours and mental welfare organizations who dealt with this problem family.

As a family doctor who has done a lot of home visits, I have seen many dirty houses, but the home of this family beggars description. Coming in through the back door (I do not think that the front door was ever used) one had to be very careful not to trip over the many pots and pans standing on the floor and not to slip on the greasy remnants of food, mixed up with heaps of dirty clothes for the wash, which evidently was always overdue. The smell was disgusting and it was advisable to hold one's breath. Yet this family was not poor at all.

It is surprising that the occurrence of skin disorders, though almost all septic, was not still greater than is indicated in chart 19a, but Mrs. Orchid did have puerperal fever after one, and abscesses of her breast after three of her deliveries. The diagram of the incidence of mental disorders (chart 19b) shows that there seems to have been little trouble in the first years. The father was the first to have nervous symptoms, due to the continual quarrels with his brother. After him his wife started, at first also due to quarrels with her mother- and sister-in-law. After some time it became apparent to me that things were more complicated in her case. It had struck me already, when I once made a home visit, that she behaved and spoke as if she were married to her unmarried brother-in-law, who was more educated than her husband. Later a neighbour told me, with tears in her eyes, that she had caught her husband in the barn, making love to Mrs. Orchid.

So I suspected that she was dissatisfied with her husband and this opinion was confirmed in subsequent home visits, when Mr. Orchid gave the impression of being completely uninterested in his wife, while I am afraid he gave more attention to his cows. Still later, Mrs. Orchid had several abortions, which she tried to conceal, and she herself then told me that she was having intercourse with another man. She wanted another baby, but at the same time she asked for the pill. She often presented with hard and swollen labia showing lacerations due to continual scratching of her vulva. There is no doubt whatever that her marriage was unsatisfactory. But the way in which this was to find expression in the relations and interactions within her family, has been appalling.

It struck me first in 1962 that something strange was happening with the children when I was told that Peter, the second boy, was "holy". At first I could not believe my ears, but it appeared that the family qas absolutely convinced of his holiness, and Mrs. Orchid told me several incidents to prove this, such as his having rescued a small child from a road accident, his kind attention and politeness, always doing things for others, his praying and his constant role of peacemaking. He came to me in the same year with several nervous symptoms, headaches and bizarre symptoms, and when later he developed a high fever due to tonsillitis, I witnessed his religious ecstasies when he was delirious.

At that time I did not yet know that "the holy child" is a recognized phenomenon in family therapy, signifying underlying marital disharmony, which "the holy child" tries to soothe and I think it most unlikely that this family had ever heard of this. This holy boy gave the family a lot of trouble later, but in 1968 he came to me again with nervous symptoms, which arose from tensions between him and his elder brother whom he detested. Next year he thought he had an eye disease, of which I

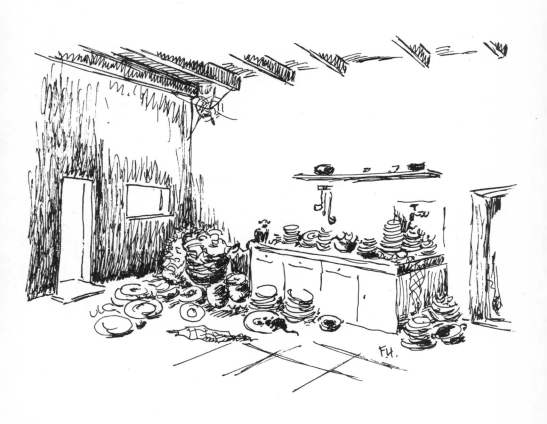

could find no signs and in 1970 he attempted suicide with sleeping tablets and had to be admitted to hospital. The reason was that he wanted to get engaged to a girl from another village (who also came from a known problem family), of whom his father disapproved, giving rise to heated family conflicts. The psychiatrist described him in the hospital discharge report as an adolescent with a badly integrated personality structure. During the next few years he became involved with homosexual relations, particularly of a triangular nature. His family, his father especially, strongly disapproved of this, giving rise to endless struggles. The "holy boy" now became the black sheep, the scapegoat of the family, another recognized phenomenon of family dynamics, also usually symptomatic of concealed marital disharmony. He has left the family, lives now in lodgings and has become a waiter. He twice again had to be admitted to a psychiatric hospital, the last time after attempting suicide due to a broken off relationship.

Events with his elder brother Alfred were still more dramatic. In 1964 his mother came with him to the surgery, saying that she thought he looked poorly and that he had no appetite. He did nothing but read and watch the T.V. I examined him and could find nothing wrong physically. In 1968 she told me that he had no friends and always stayed at home, weeping if she went away. The following year I found that she was still washing this boy of seventeen. He wanted to stay close to her and ate only if he could sit beside her. In 1970 I noted that this boy of eighteen still sat (literally) on his mother's lap and wanted to be caressed by her. He was then examined by a psychologist of the mental health organization, who phoned me afterwards and thought his intelligence was satisfactory but there was a wide gap between fantasy and reality. He looked upon his father as some kind of Santa Claus, with whom he had no opportunities to identify himself. This boy was going to study at the university, but the psychologist spoke of the poor prognosis. Psychotherapy was urgently needed, but neither mother nor son were motivated for this, thinking help to be unnecessary.

Alfred did go to university but after a year he failed and went to work in an office. In 1971 I noted that he was still being washed by his mother. In that year he began to strike and kick her, having rows at home and becoming solitary. He grew nervous and tense, being very isolated. In 1972 he did military service, but during one leave came to me and asked to be referred to a plastic surgeon, thinking that his face (in fact very handsome) must be the reason why the other boys were always teasing him. Instead of referring him, I wrote a letter to his military medical officer, but Alfred went directly to the surgeon, who wrote to me stating that it would be criminal to operate on such a face.

Still Alfred returned to me again and again. It is almost unbelievable that he was considered fit to be able to complete his military service, but he managed to do so, not wishing to be invalided on psychiatric grounds.

However, after finishing his military service he did not go back to the office, but went instead to an (also odd) farmer's family in the neighbourhood, where he worked a little and lived in. His delusions grew worse, he thought people were spying on him via the radio and in 1974 he had to be admitted to a mental hospital with overt schizophrenic symptoms. Recently his mother went to fetch him, against medical advice, and brought him home and I wonder how things will finally end.

In my opinion, this story very vividly illustrates the interactions at work in a family with repressed marital disharmony. I have never heard of open conflict between Mr. and Mrs. Orchid; other dynamic mechanisms were called for to try to keep the family in balance. I think it is evident that these had a very deleterious effect on the children. At the same time we should not overlook the fact that the ancestors of these parents were known to have been strange.

Having ended my chapter on problem families with these three medical family histories, I realize that I have made a choice. There are many problem families in my practice, at all social levels, and presenting different types of behaviour. I did not choose for example an accident-prone family, where one member after the other suffers from serious "unfortunate" events, fractures and other mishaps, which in my experience, often are associated with marital disharmony and alcoholism.

If a family doctor practises long enough to get to know his families very well, I suspect he will always be astonished by the many problems in these "normal" families. Then he will realize the truth of the words of Tolstoy, that great observer of family life: "all happy families are alike; every unhappy family is unhappy in its own way" (Anna Karenina I,1).

IX. Childless Couples

A.   Both Mr. Primrose and his wife were descended from one of the hundred older families, described in chapter XII. He came from a family with eight children and she from a family of eleven. I knew both of them from childhood. He was the son of a nursery gardener, but he went to work at the post office and married in the spring of 1956 (chart 20, appendix 2). During my summer holidays of that year my locum treated Mrs. Primrose for an infection of her right labium accompanied by a lymphadenitis in her right groin. In October she came to my surgery with nervous symptoms and when I casually made enquiries about her marriage life she burst into tears telling me that things were not as she had hoped them to be, intercourse being very painful. She longed for children, but when I examined her I found her to have vaginismus which made it difficult to palpate bimanually her small uterus. Not only her womb with a long pointed cervix but the whole girl showed signs of being infantile. I invited her husband for an interview and tried to instruct him in the art of making love to his wife. But the next year she told me that things had not improved and her nervous symptoms persisted. When they had been married for two years without her becoming pregnant I asked her to make a basal temperature chart over some months, and when this showed no evidence of ovulation I referred her to a gynaecologist, who confirmed my findings. He extended the investigation by cytology, culture (excluding tubercle bacilli) and insufflation. The husband's semen proved to be normal and there were no signs of cervical hostility, so he wrote stating he was unable to find a cause for the infertility and certainly no indication for any rational therapy. Nevertheless he prescribed hormones for her and kept making follow-up appointments until in May 1960 she came to me stating that she refused to submit herself any longer to endless examinations by the gynaecologist and his juniors.

In December 1962 we spoke again about her infertility problems which still caused her so much unhappiness. She had a strong desire for children and stated that intercourse was normal now. In 1963 she presented with vaginal discharge, caused by candida. She had been working in a kindergarten, but after a short time she had been dismissed for fondling the children too much and this distressed her.

72

When she had been married for ten years I found that she still had vaginismus. Her periods were very short, but her basal temperature curve was now definitely biphasic. I mentioned the possibility of adoption but her husband did not like this idea. At her request I referred her to a second gynaecologist, who admitted her to hospital but could find nothing abnormal, although he had doubts about the frequency of intercourse. He also spoke about adoption which they would not consider. In 1969 she wanted to be referred to a Professor in gynaecology, who diagnosed oligospermia. After a long interview with both partners, regarding the pro's and con's at their age, they desisted from further investigations. Mrs. Primrose was bitterly disappointed over her childlessness but her nervous symptoms have disappeared.

Mr. Primrose seems to have devoted himself to sport. I have seen him at least eight times for serious football-accidents, ankle sprains, a rib fracture, concussion and lastly in 1973 a ruptured meniscus of his right knee. We have spoken of their infertility problem on several occasions, but looking back I have serious doubts about the efficacy of my management. I strongly suspect that they have never had satisfactory intercourse and I am afraid that I did not focus sufficiently on this symptom. I regret this all the more as he has a brother, also a postman, whose marital history is almost exactly the same: no children, unsatisfactory and incomplete investigations leaving the same doubts about the performance of intercourse. His wife helps other households so much that she definitely seems to neglect her own husband. I think this is obvious to every one except to her and it must be an expression of a sub-conscious emotional reaction.

B.   Mrs. Rose (chart 21, appendix 2) was a stranger to me in 1950 when she entered the practice by marrying a truckdriver. He was a quiet boy whose family I knew well.

Young Mrs. Rose came to me when she had been married for ten months. Her periods were regular but she had noticed that her stomach was enlarged. To her disappointment this proved to be due to subcutaneous fat, her uterus being normal. She was very nervous and started to cry. When she had been married two years I examined her more fully. The basal temperature curve was biphasic, but the Sims-Huhner test during ovulation time showed no mobile spermatozoa and only leucocytes in the servical canal. The gynaecologist to whom I referred her did many investigations in the next two years, even operating upon her to correct the position of her uterus. Everything appeared to be normal, including seminal analysis, and the gynaecologist was optimistic regarding the chances of pregnancy, prescribing low doses of oestrogens in the first half of the cycle. After two years of intensive investigations, Mr. Rose refused to allow his wife to be examined further. Three years later she wanted to be referred to another gynaecologist, who could find nothing abnormal and who gave similar advice. In 1959 her period was overdue for three weeks, but not, it transpired, due to pregnancy.

In 1960 a third (university) gynaecologist did extensive investigations which included hormonal studies. He found an oligospermia and many abnormal spermatozoa, the Sims-Huhner test being negative four times. I suggested the possibility of adoption but the husband refused to consider this. In 1961 she was overdue again, but the pregnancy tests were negative.

In 1962 I mentioned adoption again and this time she succeeded in persuading her husband. Now a long search for a baby started. I sought the help of a social worker, and wrote letters to all kinds of social agencies. New hope sprang in her heart and with growing chances, her nervous symptoms appeared again (see chart 21). Shortly after their copper wedding anniversary in 1963 an Amsterdam agency granted Mr. and Mrs. Rose the 8 months old child of an unmarried mother. They were very pleased with this boy, their life changed completely, but only after three years of suspense were they allowed to adopt him legally as their own son.

The child grew up a nice looking, fair boy, with the usual children's diseases and accidents. In 1965 he started to cry so heavily after a fall that he became cyanotic and suddenly stopped breathing. His mother was very frightened, applied artificial respiration and put him under the cold water tap. On my arrival I could not find anything abnormal and I postulated that the boy had had a breath-holding attack.

Two years later his parents were alarmed by his frequent falls without apparent cause. His reflexes were brisk making me decide to send him to a paediatric neurologist, who arranged an electro-encephalogram which suggested probable epilepsy. His parents were very sensible when they heard of this diagnosis. Although they were worried their behaviour towards the boy was adequate and they showed no signs of overanxiety. The boy was put on anticonvulsant medication and was kept under regular supervision. He never had fits again, only once in 1971 did his left arm show some momentary clonic contractions. I reduced his medication gradually and stopped it altogether in the spring of 1974. Although he is a bit tense and nervous I doubt whether the diagnosis of epilepsy, carrying with it such a heavy social stigma, was justified after all. In my experience as a family doctor electro-encephalograms in children may do more overall harm than good.

Mr. and Mrs. Rose are still a little worried, they are afraid for instance to let the boy go swimming. For my part I worry more about his adopted-mother, something which they do not do, as she feels fine.

Mrs. Rose's periods, which had become more and more irregular with the uncertainty of legal adoption and new nervous symptoms, stopped wholly at the unusually early age of 40, accompanied by hot flushes and menopausal acroparaesthesia. In 1966 she started to have gastro-intestinal symptoms, abdominal pains and vomiting. X-rays of gallbladder, stomach and duodenum showed no abnormalities. Her symptoms were probably due to tension arising when the chance was offered of a second child from the same social agency. The symptoms returned later, in 1968, when there was trouble with the legal adoption, and they subsided with a mild sedative. In 1969 she had nervous symptoms again. This time her 77 year old father had married a woman 35 years younger than himself. So when Mrs. Rose had abdominal symptoms again in 1970, I was not at first alarmed. A new X-ray of her gallbladder showed no stones and her blood picture was normal. But at the end of that year she began to lose weight. I ordered a new gastro-duodenal series and this time a small ulcer on the lesser curvature of the stomach was found. I put her in bed on a diet, but the pains did not disappear although the ulcer on the X-ray diminished considerably. This symptom of persistent pain made me very suspicious, so I sent her to a surgeon in the spring of 1971, who performed a large resection of the stomach. The pathologist reported evidence of an undifferentiated adenocarcinoma of the stomach with definite metastases in the lymph nodes. I am very grateful that the surgeon did not tell anything to Mr. or Mrs. Rose for at the moment of writing, 5 years after her operation, Mrs. Rose feels fine: she has put on more than 20 pounds in weight and she has no complaints at all about her health. Yet, I am afraid that the story of this second childless couple will not have the happy ending it should have following the luck in finding a child to adopt.* But you never can tell. Several of my patients with proved carcinoma of the stomach have been cured by operation, and I can remember a lady (who was also childless) who lived happily for more than 20 years after a similar operation in which the abdomen was found to be full of lymphnodes with histological evidence of involvement from her gastric carcinoma. Twice I asked the pathologist to re-examine her slides and both times he had no doubts about the correctness of his original diagnosis. She died in her sleep when she was 65, probably due to coronary infarction.

The histories of these two couples contain elements that keep returning in the history of many childless couples, i.e. coital problems, endless investigations without conclusive evidence of pathology, the distress of being childless and the wandering from doctor to doctor while the couple grows too old for adoption.

I inevitably made a selection in choosing these two examples. In 1972 the Medical Faculty of the Nijmegen University organized a symposium on childless marriage and I was asked to contribute as a family doctor, which gave me an opportunity to review the problems of childless marriages. I

* In 1977 Mrs. Rose developed a mass in the lower abdomen, which proved on operation to be a Krukenberg tumor. Despite therapy with cytostatics she died a few months after the operation. The serenity of her deathbed has highly impressed the consultants and nurses in hospital.

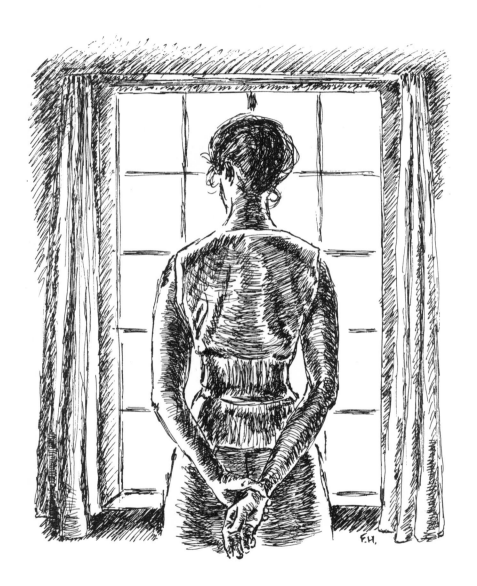

started by studying the literature, but came to the disappointing conclusion that almost all publications had been written by gynaecologists and some by psychiatrists, both based on selected case-material, while little attention was paid to the family aspects. I was not able to find comprehensive and more or less representative population studies. General practitioners, surveying their practice populations, have written remarkably little about this subject, and seem to have followed the general trend of society by neglecting the problems of childless couples. I found only two studies: the excellent article by a British general practitioner Jensen (1966) and a lecture of the Dutch general practitioner of Amsterdam, Brühl, while the Leiden Lecturer in general practice, Bremer (1974) published his article after the symposium. I was therefore more or less forced to rely on my own experience and to do a retrospective personal study about prevalence, presentation, causes and effects of childlessness.

In doing so I learned six lessons, which may be of some value to other family doctors. Generally speaking almost 10% of all marriages remain childless, the same average figure was found in the three practices associated with our Institute. I found that by far the most important factor is the age of the wife at the time of wedding, this being in general older in the countryside and in upper social levels then in the cities and in lower social classes. Ten percent of all marriages is no small figure, but I found that on the average a general practitioner is consulted by his patients only about five times a year for a new infertility problem, while he is consulted several hundreds of times a year for the undesirable problem of excessive fertility. These mere figures will make clear that a general practitioner may run the risk of underestimating the importance of the problem of barrenness, and may be in danger of not developing skills in handling such problems.

Investigating the problem I undertook a detailed study of the records of a hundred childless couples, who had been my patients for more than five years. I reached the uncomfortable conclusion that about half of them never spoke of being childless while I am convinced that the majority did not wish to remain so and that of those who did consult, most were very late in doing so, ranging from two to eight years after their wedding. There must have been a considerable barrier between my patients and me for them not to broach this subject, whilst I thought I knew my patients so well! Many of them evidently needed being met more than halfway by a sympathetic doctor who could anticipate their problems. I felt that I had failed in this which was the first lesson I learned.

The second lesson was, that many of the patients had prematurely broken off the investigations they underwent, either by me or the gynaecologist, without my realizing this sufficiently. There seems to have been a definite resistance against examination of their fertility, especially by husbands. The outcome of my study in assessing the causes of infertility was (in agreement with the three other authors) that in a considerable proportion the cause remained uncertain. Of the known causes (apart from the age of the wife) gynaecological diseases and previous operations seemed to be the most important, but these were immediately followed by sexual problems like vaginismus, impotence, homosexuality or, in short, problems in their relationship. While most of the organic causes of female and male sterility (except varicocele) were incurable, the majority of these behaviour problems might have been cured by relatively simple therapy, if started early enough before certain habits had been engrained or hope had been abandoned. The search through my notes taught me that straight forward explanations such as showing a young man how wide the vagina of his wife is, dilatation of an excessively stiff hymen and sometimes a temporary prohibition of intercourse, or simple behaviour therapy, in fact, were often followed by complete success. But all too often I had missed the opportunity when the time was there, and I failed to focus on the relationship, sticking to the "patient" who came to me, instead of inviting the couple to come together and concentrating on their interactions. That was my third lesson.

Re-reading my records and taking note of the results of an inquiry of the childless couples in our practices by the psychologist Bierkens, I was impressed by the misery and distress crying out from these documents. Both Brühl and Jensen had presented evidence which suggested that childless couples were more nervous and I thought this very probable. I even had the impression that they had more organic diseases requiring medical treatment than fertile couples had. Brühl and Jensen collected and coded their material retrospectively. Jensen looked only at the women and Brühl did not make use of controls. I had the advantage of having at my disposal the already coded morbidity data of the hundred young and older families of this book over some twenty years and of the whole practice over the last five years. I decided to do a very careful study, making use of matched controls, taking into account date of marriage, age of husband and wife, social class and type of health insurance. Our sociologist, Van Eyk, and our statistician, Gubbels, helped me to analyse the data of 43 selected couples in which we ignored the morbidity due to reproductive organs. My kind of practice enabled us to choose in several instances married brothers or sisters of the childless couples as controls to make the comparisons nearly perfect. The result of our study showed that there were no statistically significant differences between the childless and the fertile couples, neither for the women nor for the men, regarding number of consultations, referrals to specialists, admissions to hospital, number of episodes of nervous trouble or other morbidity. The apparent differences between women with and without children were directly contrary to our expectation. I learned it from my fourth lesson: in doing research one has to use strictly comparable groups with data collected and coded without the possibility of bias creepin in.

78

The negative results of this study do not allow us, of course, to draw the conclusion that childlessness is no heavy burden for the couples in question. But there are reasons to assume that the stress in having no children is matched by the stress of having children.

Couples who wish for, but do not have children, are faced with the big problem of assimilation. This is a process which needs time and in which, despite individual differences, phases can be recognized. After a shorter or longer phase of denial of the problem, the truth is gradually realized. In this second phase, the process of making decisions leading to the seeking of medical advice or not takes place with greater or lesser anguish. The third phase is the period of medical examinations, usually a disagreeable period for the couple, in which they are strongly confronted with their sexual functioning. Every menstrual period in this phase may give rise to bursts of tears. At first the general practitioner is consulted, later specialists and later still sometimes quacks. Some couples tend to shop endlessly from one doctor to another. In a following phase the possibility of never having children is acknowledged and gradually faced. The wife decides to accept or to continue a job. In a final phase the couple accepts the fact and is able to resign themselves to it and to detach themselves from the problem; the advantages of staying childless can also be realized.

It is evident that there are great individual variations between couples in the process of working through their problems, but it also became evident to me, when I re-read my records of childless couples, that although many needed support and advice to be able to master their problem, in a number of cases I had failed to give sufficient or correct support in the right phase. Thus I learned my fifth lesson: a family doctor needs some knowledge of the phases of this process and of the help that can be needed in each of them, although the ability to listen with a sensitive mind and an accurate empathetic understanding are the most important requirements.

My sixth and last lesson was of a more comforting nature: many originally childless couples appear to have had children without any or with only placebo therapy, sometimes after many years and sometimes despite a very poor prognosis by the gynaecologist. Therefore I think that a certain optimism seems to be justified when confronted with childlessness.

References:
Bierkens, P.B. (1973), Ned. T. Geneesk. 117, 770-776.
Bremer, G.J. (1974), Kinderloosheid in de huisartspraktijk, Huisarts en Wetenschap, 17, 85-92.
Jensen, P. (1966), J. Coll. Gen. Pract. II, 150-165.

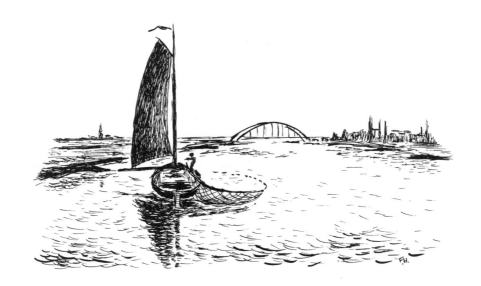

X. Families with a Chronic Patient

1. A Father with a Chronic Illness

Mr. Snowdrop (chart 22, appendix 2) was a fisherman living in an old brick house on the riverside, with two very old lime trees in front pruned in the shape of two enormous candelabras. When the town was bombarded in 1943, he was there and witnessed how many were killed in his immediate vicinity. It was then that he stopped working and that his illness started: a tic douloureux of the left facial nerve due to a trigeminal neuralgia. Seven years before he had had a Bell's paralysis on the same side with ensuing long lasting disability. He also had chronic bronchitis. I referred him to a neurologist, who prescribed medicine and galvanic treatment first, and afterwards admitted him to hospital, where the neurosurgeon did the Spiller-Fraiser operation, the second and third branch of his trigeminal nerve being cut through. At first there was a complete anaesthesia of the corresponding region, but after some months paraesthesia followed and the next year the same agonizing pains returned together with spasms in his left facial muscles. He felt very weak, developed a tendency to collapse with diarrhoea, his gait was ataxic and he was very thin. I have never been able to understand his illness completely, neither could the neurologist nor the neurosurgeon. In 1946 he was admitted to hospital again where the possibility of a tumour of the acoustic nerve was ruled out. An intracranial complication seemed however very likely, probably a chronic inflammation of the pia arachnoid with scarring. In the following years pain spread to his left knee and shoulder, he became deaf in his left ear. But at the same time it became gradually clear, that a considerable proportion of his more and more dramatic complaints were of nervous origin and had an hysterical character. He visited several quacks, as orthodox medicine appeared to be unable to help him. Things grew worse and worse and he started to tyrannize his family and neighbours, sending panic messages to me at the most impossible times. It struck me time and again, that he presented his symptoms as if they were quite new, while in reality he had been complaining of them for many years. The neurologist gave local suboccipital hydrocortison injections, and later the neurosurgeon did a nerve evulsion, but no benefit ensued. Medical treatment proved to be of no help and I came to the conclusion that the only thing which brought about temporary relief were distractive measures. His family told me that striking improvements took place if he had interesting visitors or when he could play cards. All his symptoms would then disappear suddenly. This made his eldest son disbelieve the intensity of his father's complaints, leading to nasty family quarrels, and resulting in this son leaving the family. Mr. Snowdrop took to bed for long periods, but with symptomatic and distractive measures I succeeded in mobilizing him again and again. He even started to run some errands and to do some work in his garden. In the beginning of the sixties things deteriorated: he upset people, urinated in the livingroom, wet his son's bed and even drank his own urine. He often said pathetically that he longed for his death but at the same time it was apparent that the thought terrified him. In 1962 he grew calmer, although complaining bitterly that his wife was neglecting him, while in fact she was spoiling him. It was a relief (though no one dared to say so then) when he was found dead in his bed one morning at the age of 74 in 1963.

I am sure that he had an organic illness, but I am also sure that his clinical picture was highly coloured by hysterical reactions, it being absolutely impossible to distinguish between these two components. Every general practitioner will have one or two similar patients in his practice, keeping him in constant doubt and making treatment very difficult. I have doubts after all about the wisdom of referring Mr. Snowdrop to the neurosurgeon, as it seems highly probable that the progressive intracranial scarring was due to the Spiller-Fraiser operation. Unintentionally we produce a lot of iatrogenic harm, and I sometimes wonder if the side effects of our endeavours do not outweigh the benefits.

Mr. Snowdrop's illness had a serious impact on his family. When we look at the chart of the medical history of this family we see in the beginning that his wife was seldom ill. In 1949 she developed vaginal prolapse and I gave her a pessary which I changed regularly. She never complained about her husband's behaviour, but in November 1952 I was called because she felt dizzy and weak. Her faeces were black and her haemoglobin was only 30%. I sent her to hospital, where a duodenal ulcer was confirmed. She did not want an operation and came home in December. In 1953 she had a pyelitis — her prolapse having disappeared — in 1957 a bronchopneumonia and in 1958 again a severe gastric bleed. I had to visit her in hospital several times to convince her she needed an operation, which revealed one gastric and two duodenal ulcers. In 1959 she began to have nervous symptoms, which worsened in 1961. At that time her husband was very difficult, and friction had arisen between her and her future daughter-in-law who had come to live in the house which was going to be rebuilt. Her son sided with his fiancée and mother felt excluded. During my visits in those days, husband and wife competed in complaining; both of them sought my ear for their laments, but neither of them seemed to hear what the other was saying, an

82

almost humorous performance. I introduced our social worker who found out that Mrs. Snowdrop was really worried lest she be pushed aside. The son had bought the house and in the plans for re-building no room was reserved for her while it was impossible for her to sleep with her husband. Things were rearranged, the daughter-in-law returned to her parents and better plans were made in peace. The chart shows how her medical demands diminished almost dramatically in 1962. In the last year of her husband's life, some nervous symptoms reappeared which disappeared completely after his death never to return again. She developed severe hypertension in 1966, which proved impossible to control. Her daughter-in-law told me that she took to drinking in 1970, having four or five bottles of cognac a week. In the evenings she often stumbled and fell. She felt lonely and useless and in the autumn of that year she went into a home for old people.

The two sons developed differently. The youngest son is rather dull with no enterprise, and is still a house-painter's help. He turned the old house into a bungalow and married a girl of a low social class. The eldest son is extremely intelligent. He worked himself up as a broker, entered higher social circles, married a well-to-do girl and built a very fine house in a different village but also on the riverside. He always tried to defend his mother and seemed to detest his father. I wonder whether this has something to do with his sexual development for it has become obvious that he is a homosexual.

2. *A Mother with a Chronic Illness*

Mrs. Tulip (chart 23, appendix 2) was married to a small business man. They had six children and they both worked hard. It was an extremely nice sound family, always cheerful and with a pleasant atmosphere in the house, which everybody liked to visit. They were not greatly ambitious for themselves and they were always ready to help others. The youngest boy was born eight years after his elder brother and when Mrs. Tulip was pregnant with him her illness became apparent: she had an essential hypertension. What shall I say of her medical history? Every doctor will know the likelihood of events that followed in the days before we had really potent weapons to control blood pressure.

In 1946 her tension was 230/130 and it stayed so for years. She was practically without symptoms and it was difficult to convince her she needed treatment. In 1949 she had thrombophlebitis in her varicose veins and perhaps it is relevant to mention that she had a mobile swelling in her right groin, growing and diminishing in size with her periods, probably due to endometriosis. In 1952 she had her first varicose ulcer and in the same year she had her first attack of cardiac asthma. Her blood pressure rose to 250/140 and she had to be digitalized. In 1953 she had her second attack after she had stopped taking her tablets and her second varicose ulcer took two months to heal. The treatment of the hypertension caused her more symptoms than the disease itself — as is usual — and this made her frequently fail to stick to her regime, which she had to pay for with noctural dyspnoes. In 1955 she began to walk with difficulty due to arthritis of the knees (she was as might be anticipated far too heavy), and this worsened during the following years.

In 1957 she had her first attack of cerebral palsy, from which she recovered reasonably well. After the second attack however her gait was much worse. She aged unusually rapidly and had the greatest difficulty in climbing stairs. In 1958 she was unable to walk even a few paces. It was an interesting observation that her tension fell then and remained practically normal, being systolic 170/150, diastolic 90. The family let me into their secret; she was now unable to lay her hands on salt, something she had always done behind my back. In 1959 the blood urea began to rise and in 1960 she had a myocardial infarction after which she developed atrial fibrillation. She started to vomit, lost weight and became extremely anaemic. In september 1961 she suddenly died while going to bed, probably due to a second coronary infarction. She was then 57 years old and in her last years her blood pressure had always stayed within normal limits 140/80.

A mother's chronic illness, especially of a large family like Mrs. Tulip's has serious consequences for the family. Somebody has to help and gradually take over the housekeeping. Usually this is one of the daughters and often, as in this case, the youngest daughter stays at home as a Cinderella, her best years passing by.

I have seen this happen often and usually these girls became somewhat sour. But I must say that I have seldom seen a girl so cheerful, sound and noble as Mrs. Tulip's second daughter. She has had an enormous burden to carry. She still looks after her father, but the chart shows that she hardly ever needed medical help. The consultations she sought were for measles, wax in her ear seven times, small accidents, a cold, primrose dermatitis and only once for sleeping problems. We also see that nervous symptoms have been remarkebly rare in the whole family. Yet there has been enough serious disease: the father has diabetes (he usually tests his own urine) and has been operated upon for cholecystitis with stones, the second son had chronic osteomyelitis that flares up, a serious lobar pneumonia, a herpes zoster, bronchitis and several other respiratory infections. The eldest daughter had typhoid fever in 1951, a fractured leg in 1954, erythema nodosum in 1956 due to Boeck's disease becoming apparent in 1957.

On re-reading what I have just written about family Tulip, I suppose it will be evident to my readers that I have sympathy with, and even admiration for, this family and indeed I consider this to be a sound and wholesome family, able to cope with the most serious difficulties. I have paid it so many visits in all kind of circumstances, seeing and sensing how they lived together. These visits stopped after Mrs. Tulip's death and I did not see much of them. When I heard in 1963 that Mr. Tulip was going to re-marry I was glad and pleased as I thought that he merited this. He knew his second wife well; two of his sons had married two of her daughters. The second Mrs. Tulip was a widow, running a business elsewhere and in the first months of their marriage they lived in her house. After closing her business in 1965 she came to live in his house. When she came to see me with her husband at the end of July, I got the impression that they were very well matched. She told me that she had undergone a cholecystectomy for gall stones eight month's previously and a hysterectomy for menorrhagia, four months previously. She had pains in her lower abdomen now, feeling some pressure on her bladder and anus. I examined her and within a few minutes I realized that yet another drama was developing within this family, as I found her vaginal walls to be infiltrated, with a hard swelling in the pouch of Douglas. A phone call to the gynaecologist who had operated on her confirmed my fears; she had a cervical carcinoma, possibly complicated by a secondary infection. Within a few days she ran a high fever and had to stay in bed. She had to endure horrible suffering before she died: high fever, agonizing pains, nausea, thrombosis, and an extreme anaemia. Soon I had to start morphia injections and at first it seemed likely that her end would not be far off. I visited her in the mornings and also late every night, to talk with her and to give her an injection to make sleep possible. When she seemed ready for it I gradually told her the truth. It took an exceptionally long time before she began to accept it, because at the same time she did not really want to know what was going on. In the evenings we could talk about the nature of her disease and the prognosis in such a way that her husband and I had no doubts whatsoever that she understood very well what was going to happen, even giving me the feeling that we had an intense contact, while the next morning she could ask "when will I get better, doctor?" Several times she was all but moribund, but evaded death in an almost miraculous way, seeming to fight and resist death till the bitter end. But she was only 53 and had just started a new life. It is no wonder that this time both husband and her step-daughter — who again looked after this patient — developed sleeping problems, when at last the mercy of death had taken her away.

Mr. Tulip appears to have been born without luck. Yet for all that he seems to me to be a happy man and I know him rather well, observing for instance his behaviour when he himself was dangerously ill and had his operation a few months ago. I think he has always had a certain basic contentment within himself reinforced by his religious attitude to life.

I have witnessed the process of dying in hundreds of families. At first I paid my visits to these families reluctantly and I detected a tendency to postpone or forget these visits. But soon I came to learn the very rewarding character of caring for the dying. A family doctor can be of great importance to those who are going to die and to their families, not only in what he does, but also in his being a reliable and understanding bystander. I have seen men and women and their families rise to the challenge as a climax of human existence. But it is hazardous to predict who will stand up to this final test: some religious and educated people will fail and some simple souls, or those who are thought to have lost their religious beliefs, will succeed.

Rereading this chapter in 1978 I can add that my prediction was right as far as concerns Mr. Tulip. He proved to have a carcinoma of the oesophagus which could not be removed in time. He refused to have symptomatic operations and last year he died like a hero, kindly looked after in his home by his daughter, enjoying the sun and the look of the river till his last hours.

3. *A Family with a Handicapped Child*

Mrs. Violet's obstetrical history is a very instructive one — at least it was to me. She became pregnant shortly after her marriage in 1950 (chart 24, appendix 2) and everything seemed perfectly normal at her regular antenatal check-ups, till she started to have labour pains a month before her time. She had no loss of blood and the cervix was closed. I ordered her to stay in bed. The foetal heart sounds were audible and normal, but next day these had disappeared and she did not feel foetal movements anymore. The following day she was delivered in a very short time of a macerated still-born child 51 cm long, weighing 1900 gram. The placenta was large and flat, showing dark blood clots on the maternal side. I took foetus and placenta to the pathologist but he found only signs of foetal asphyxia, the placenta being normal on microscopic examination. The blood pressure of Mrs. Violet had never been higher than 130/80 while her urine had always been normal.

Within a few months she was pregnant for the second time. Again everything appeared to be normal till the end of her seventh month, when she suddenly got abdominal pains while she was straining on her stools. She was restless and her uterus felt hard while the foetal heart could no longer be heard. this time the blood pressure was 140/110. The cervix was still closed, I gave her a morphia injection and in the evening a still-born foetus was born within intact membranes filled with blood, together with a small placenta full of dark clots, the typical picture of abruptio placentae. I made a note in red ink on her record to prescribe a strict saltfree diet and bed rest from the beginning, in the event of a following pregnancy. This I did and a full term healthy boy resulted from this next pregnancy. In her fifth pregnancy the blood pressure rose progressively, making it necessary to induce labour at eight months. The delivery took place rapidly and the child, this time a girl, was born within the membranes, delivered simultaneously with the placenta which showed many white hard infarcted nodules. During the night after her birth this small girl developed signs of an intracranial haemorrhage and had to be admitted to hospital. When she came home, she was far better than I had expected her to be, but seeing her two months later in the baby clinic, it struck me on examination that she had a white visual reflex on both eyes. The ophthalmologist to whom I referred her confirmed total congenital cataract, for which he advised an operation when she would be one year old. This was done and although the eye surgeon was enthusiastic about the results I do not think that the girl has ever been able to see anything. Intensive investigations by the paediatrician revealed no cause for her cataract and the electro-encephalogram was normal. Ann did not at first give the impression of being backward, indeed she was a lively child. But with the progress of time it became evident that her development was retarded; she never learned to sit and she never spoke a word. All day she was busy with herself, her movements being athetoid. In August 1960 she developed fits and had again to be admitted to hospital where the paediatrician felt they were secondary to pneumonia in both lower lungs. With Bobath physio-therapy, continued after her discharge, she improved. While in hospital Ann was able to eat everything, but returning home her mother said that as before she would only take sieved food. The physiotherapist, who saw her regularly told me that occasionallly her right arm showed clonic contractions, while her face would get red and she would cry afterwards, suggestive of larval fits, which disappeared after I prescribed phenobarbitone. Ann was admitted to hospital several times afterwards, mostly for her eyes, while she was also seen regularly by the pediatrician. She got buphthalmos and made absolutely no progress in her mental development, growing only in length. It was a shocking sight to see this blind and idiotic child lying in her cot, with her legs sticking out between the bars, uttering only loud and fierce inhuman cries. She could only be kept quiet by having the radio playing continuously. At times I suggested her admission to an institution, but her parents declined. I visited them regularly. Ann kept on growing with her food always ground in the mixer. She became far too heavy to be carried by her mother and her father had to come home several times a day to help. At last she was almost as tall as her mother, her breasts developed and she started to menstruate. At that time her mother was ready for Ann's admission, but her father would still not hear of it. It proved to be impossible for Mrs. Violet or for her family to discuss this matter with him, as he gave no comment. Each of my visits to her and Ann ended with her hopeless sobbing. After having tried several times to talk things over with Mr. Violet, without much success, I decided to use a medical argument; Mrs. Violet's blood pressure was going up again and I told her husband that this made it unjustifiable to keep Ann at home any longer. Mr. Violet was a reasonable man but he was deeply attached to his daughter. He argued for some time, arranged at first for a home-help for his wife, but at last he gave in. I think that the decisive argument which finally convinced him was that it would be better for Ann herself. It proved to be possible to send Ann to an institution for a holiday, and this made it evident to both parents that she could equally well be cared for by others and their doubts and fears disappeared. Still it took a long time to find a permanent place in an institution, achieving success in 1969 when Ann was almost 12 years old. Both parents are happy with this situation now, the father still brings small presents to me as he always did while I was looking after his daughter.

Mrs. Violet's blood pressure has returned to normal with only reserpine, although she was on the pill. Yet it is evident that she is a high risk for vascular complications; her mother died of a cerebral vascular accident, her father had angina pectoris, a necrotic toe and became blind, due to vascular lesions in his occipital lobe. One of her brothers had to be operated on for intermittent claudication and two others had myocardial infarctions.

Ann's disease has certainly had an effect on her mother's health and a look at the chart makes it highly probable that this also applies to her father. It is true that, before he got married, he twice had a duodenal ulcer, but this recurred in 1958, after Ann's birth. This time lengthy bedrest and diet brought no relief, so that at last he needed surgery, revealing an almost healed ulcer on the back and a fresh active one on the front of his duodenum. But this operation brought no relief; he developed a peptic ulcer of his jejunum which took a very long time to heal. During the time of waiting for Ann's admission to the mental institution, he had a humeroscapular periarthritis which was resistant to therapy, leading to a frozen shoulder, but all these symptoms disappeared quite unexpectedly after Ann's admission, as did also his gastric troubles necessitating no further operation and now he is able to tolerate all kinds of food and drink.

I have no doubt that Ann's presence influenced unfavourably the development of her two brothers. There was no room for them in their home for Ann monopolized their parents completely. She filled the whole living-room with her cries and the constant sound of the radio. On my visits I saw only glimpses of her brothers, silently retiring to the kitchen or upstairs. They never had friends and behaved quietly and unobtrusively. The eldest developed bad posture, a round back and sloping shoulders, looking as if he wanted to conceal himself, while years of intensive physio-therapy did not improve this. Both boys had periods of nervous symptoms in the guise of stomach aches, headaches and both had trouble at school.

There has not been much research done about the impact on the family of chronic illness of one of its members. It is evident that illness of the father endangers the social-economic level of the family, though this was more obvious before the establishment of state social security. There is often an exchange in social role-components between husband and wife and for the children (especially for boys) the opportunity to have someone around with whom they can identify is decreased.

88

With chronic illness of the mother, as well as interfering with the family's sexual and reproductive functions, the physical and emotional caring functions are threatened.

The sociologist Philipsen (1974) did an enlightening longitudinal study of 57 families with a hydrocephalic child and found that most important problems lay in the field of daily life: isolation of the family, relative neglect of the other children and extreme lack of freedom for the mother (in 71% of the families). In 65% of the families the medical and social care gave rise to problems and in 59% the illness of the child gave rise to problems in the father's work (frequent job changes, failure to be promoted, extra earnings needed and a tendency to stay away from home), while in 53% the marriage suffered. We came across several of the problems mentioned in this paper looking back on the Violet family history.

Philipsen also found that the problems were more frequent where the child was seriously handicapped or from the lower social classes. When the child was admitted to an institution the family problems diminished, but the frequency of marriage problems increased. Another G.P., Van Es (1959) found that the social-psychological function of the family suffered most severely with the admission of the child leading to great benefit.

I will not cite other authors because it is not my intention in this book to review the literature. But it does seem to be appropriate to mention that the impact of chronic illness on the family is a promising subject for research by family doctors, combining with sociologists and psychologists.

4. A Family which needed a Chronic Patient

Mr. Water-lily was a successful business man. After the death of his first wife, when he was 45, he remarried, as he needed someone to look after his five children, who were still young. When I came into this practice his youngest son had married and lived next door, being a partner in the family firm with Mr. Water-lily and the eldest son. Mr. Water-lily's youngest daughter was also married but lived elsewhere, while his three eldest children lived with him and their step-mother. Two of them were handicapped: his second daughter Gladys was mentally handicapped and his son George suffered from epilepsy.

I had to visit the Water-lily family regularly. Almost all contacts shown in chart 25 (appendix 2) were house calls. They insisted upon this and it struck me in those first years I was not meant to look after the handicapped children, but only the second mother.

Occasionally she was really ill, when in 1944 she had diphtheria and in later years when she sometimes had bouts of bronchitis. But she did not have a serious chronic illness in those years, with the exception of a slightly elevated blood pressure and perhaps some arthritis. Still the family expected me to call regularly. I noted on my record that she herself did not seem to complain, but that everybody else in the family thought it essential that I look after her. She was a nice woman, giving a somewhat insecure impression, talking slowly and always anxiously noting the reaction of others to what she had said. She entirely spoiled her mentally handicapped step-daughter Gladys.

Mr. Water-lily developed symptoms of emphysema and heart failure in 1954 and the next year got bronchopneumonia with ensuing empyema, which I drained. When he died he was 83 years of age. His wife had herpes zoster in 1956, she developed atrial fibrillation in 1959 and the next year she suddenly died at the age of 86.

Gladys started to give trouble soon after her father's death. She refused to eat and drink, stayed in bed and wanted to die, too. The family could not manage her and it became necessary to engage a trained nurse to stay with the family and help them to cope with her problems. The nurse gradually mobilized Gladys and got her to eat, but after she departed Gladys gradually relapsed into such a deep depression that she had to be admitted to a psychiatric hospital. One would have expected to see the family breathe more easily after being relieved of Gladys' extreme demands, but the reverse in fact appeared to be true. The three of them, and even the son living nextdoor, started to have all kinds of nervous symptoms. They lost their appetite, could not sleep and began to quarrel with each other, each one blaming the other. They appeared unable to live without Gladys and took her home against the doctor's advice. The same cycle of events happened in 1958 when Gladys had to be admitted to hospital because of appendicitis.

After her step-mother died Gladys again became deeply depressed, locking herself in the toilet for days on end, weeping and crying that she also wanted to go to heaven. Again a nurse was engaged, but this one failed to cope with the situation and fled from the family after a fortnight. Nothing has changed essentially in this family since then. They are all constantly complaining to me about each other. They cannot live together, but at the same time they cannot do without one another. In this family a pathological equilibrium has been established. It seems to need a chronic patient to stabilize its internal conflicts and tensions. They blame one another for spoiling Gladys but all of them collude in this, including the married brother. He is head of the firm now and I have the impression that he spends more time with his sisters and brother than with his wife.

Gladys is very backward indeed, but she well realizes her power over the family, exploiting it to the utmost. She has grown very fat, although she never eats with the family; she insists that special meals be prepared for her at the most impossible hours. All her whims, even the most extravagant ones, are immediately obeyed by the family. She stays in bed till after mid-day, except on days when she thinks that I might visit her, because she knows that I do not approve of her staying in bed so long. I am the only person who has any power over her. Yet I realize that I have become a part of this family system and that I assist in maintaining its pathological balance. My authority is called on only when they think it is useful for their purposes. They phone me very often and even now in 1978 I find I have to visit them at least once a month to let them talk about their problems, which are always the same. I am unhappy with this state of affairs, but I have not been able to bring about any real change for the better in this family; it has gone on in the same way for years and years. I twice introduced social workers, but neither of them succeeded in bringing about any alterations. The members of this family are completely trapped in their ambiguous mutual bonds.

Combined family therapy could help them to free themselves and I suggested this to them. After a considerable period of hesitation they made an appointment with our family therapist, but they postponed it several times and finally cancelled it indefinitely. I am afraid that I shall have to continue accepting them as they are as long as this family exists.

This story of the Water-lily family illustrates another mechanism in family dynamics; some families need a chronic patient to be able to continue their existence. In my opinion this chapter about families with a chronic patient would not have been complete without an example of this curious phenomenon.

References:
Es, J.C. van (1959), Gezinnen met zwakzinnige kinderen, Van Gorcum & Comp., Assen.
Philipsen, H. (1974), Nederlands Tijdschrift voor Geneeskunde, 118, 885-886.

PART II: FAMILY SURVEYS

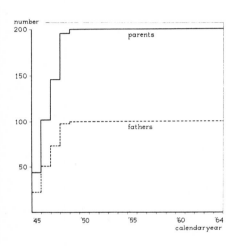

Fig. 4. Recruitement of 100 younger families

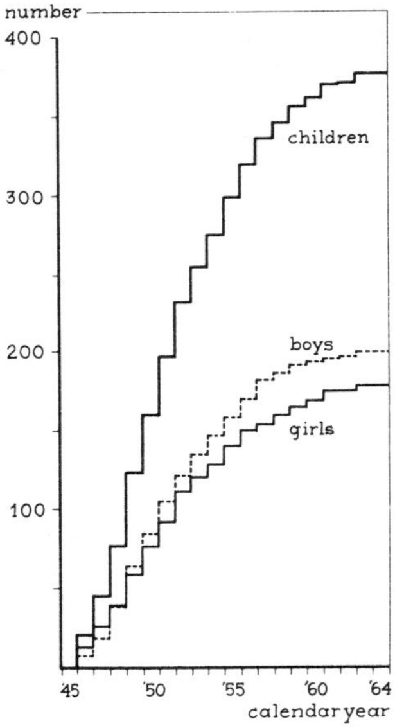

Fig. 5. The arrival of children in 100 younger families

opposite

XI. A Hundred Younger Families

Introduction

So far in this book I have only described case-histories. After having studied the medical life history of some dozens of individual families, however, I felt this approach had limitations: no generalizations or conclusions could be drawn, because it represents a selection. Accordingly I surveyed a random sample of a hundred younger and a hundred older families in my practice as I mentioned earlier in the introduction to this book. My practice comprised then practically the entire population of three urban villages.

In this chapter I will describe some results of the survey I did in 1965 of one hundred younger families. The period of observation was begun in 1945 and extended to 1965. As it was necessary to cover the medical history of these families from its beginning, I took the records of all those in the practice who married in 1945 and added successively all who married in each of the following years till I reached a total of 100 families. Fig. 4 and 5 will make it clear how the population built up in the observation period, as successively almost 400 children were born, only 14 couples having no children. Overall more than 8000 patient-years were recorded. The medical records of these families were carefully scrutinized with all diagnoses, consultations, emergency consultations, referrals to specialists and admissions to hospital being coded. In addition to the medical data, psycho-social data was collected in 1965 by the domiciliary health-team of two family doctors then working in this practice, our doctor's assistant (who in Holland combines the functions of a receptionist and nurse), the district nurse (who in Holland combines this function with those of the British health visitor) and the social worker. My partner dr. Thom van Thiel worked with me for several years, my doctor's assistant, miss Emmy van de Ven, for fifteen years and the district nurse for some ten years. All of us knew these families well although the social worker appeared to be acquainted with only a small proportion of the families.

To classify morbidity we used the E(imerl) list published by the Royal College of General Practitioners. I devised my own system to group these diagnoses together in some broader categories as described already in chapter I. The hundred young families were coded by Van Thiel and the hundred older families by myself. At that time we used the same coding system in our day to day practice, which made us have daily discussions over our criteria. For that reason I do not think that there can be much difference between our ways of classification. It was dr. Van Thiel's intention to write a thesis about the hundred young families, but his departure to begin his own practice elsewhere prevented him from achieving this.

As most of the psycho-social characteristics were based on subjective judgments of the domiciliary team we proceeded as follows. Each of us scored his judgment of the families individually, using criteria, derived from the relevant literature, we had agreed upon on beforehand. Our scores were compared in a combined meeting with the sociologist, psychologist and social worker of the Institute of Social Medicine. When there was agreement there was no problem. When the scores differed markedly we had to defend our opinions in debate and the final score was made by the independent experts. We tried to assess qualities like intelligence and neurotic instability of the parents, their marriage relationship, the parent-child relationship, the ability of the mother to care for her children and the house, hygiene, housing, finances and social contacts of the family, and we tried to measure the burden the families had to carry, such as lodgers and other social factors. This data was punched out on cards and fed to a computer.

Objects of this study

The analysis of this wealth of material offered several possibilities. Three main aims in doing this study were:
1. to demonstrate relationships that could be used in the instruction of medical students e.g.: the relationship between sex and age and different diseases,
2. to find evidence to support the thesis, as discussed in earlier chapters, that a family doctor should consider the family as a integral unit of its own,
3. to find out important relationships between the medical and social data of the families.

Results

It is not my intention in this book to become involved in a detailed account of the statistical analysis we undertook. Instead I hope to present some of the most important conclusions in a readable shape. But for readers interested in statistics or details, tables will be found in appendix I. Table XI,1 gives an account of the most important basic data of the population observed.

Our study provided considerable material, useful for teaching medical students. Fig. 6 gives an example of the incidence of respiratory tract

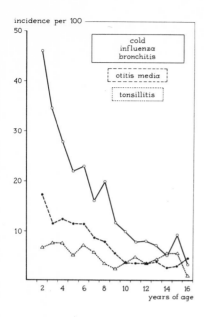

Fig. 6. Age incidence of some respiratory disorders in 100 younger families.

infections in the children. "Vertical" (descending) respiratory infections such as the common cold, influenza-like diseases, bronchitis and pneumonia were much more age-dependent than an "horizontal" respiratory infection like tonsillitis, while otitis media takes an intermediate position between these two. This has already been demonstrated in the thousand family study of Miller e.a. (1960) in Newcastle upon Tyne. Fig. 7 shows that septic skin conditions were both more frequent and more age-dependent than allergic skin conditions. Accidents and nervous dis-

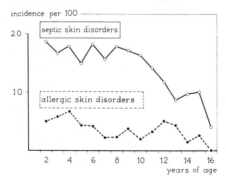

Fig. 7. Age incidence of septic and allergic skin disorders in children of the 100 younger families.

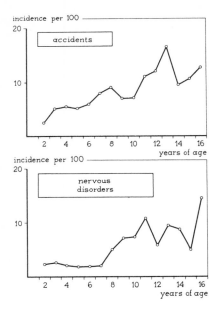

Fig. 8. Age incidence of accidents (upper) and nervous disorders (lower) in children of the 100 younger families.

orders (fig. 8) showed a definite increase in frequency as children grew older. This increase makes it very likely indeed that the incidence of this kind of symptom has a relationship with children gradually entering the world outside the family. I will give only these four examples of our epidemiological findings as they generally were in accordance with those of Hodgkin (1973) and Fry (1974), who wrote excellent books about common diseases of individuals in general practice. I prefer for the purposes of this book to concentrate on our findings concerning the family.

The figures for diagnoses and consultations were linked to individual family members. This made it possible to investigate the relationships of frequency of illnesses within the family. The Nijmegen University statistical department computed indices for the fathers, mothers and children (taken together per family) and tested the relationships between these by computing degrees of correlation (see table XI,2 appendix 1).

There proved to be statistically significant relationships, especially between parents and children, the degree of correlation being greatest between mothers and children. We can conclude that the computer results support the assumption that the family had to be regarded as a unit. There appeared to be a certain "familiality" of illness.

After this first step we looked at the distribution of illness in the families over the whole observation period. Did the families, or its members, who were often (or seldom) ill at the beginning of this period tend to continue

98

this characteristic in the following years? To study this we divided the whole span of observation into four consecutive periods of four years (ignoring the year of marriage as this was often only partially documented). We applied Friedman's method to assess agreement between the 100 families in order of numbers of diagnoses and consultations over these four periods.

Table XI,3 (appendix 1) makes it clear that there is not the slightest doubt that there was consistency over the years in the presentation of illness to their family doctor by these families. This consistency was shown by fathers, mothers, children (taken together per family) and most of all, by families as a unit.

We also looked at the relationships between totals of diagnoses and consultations per year for each of these periods, (see table XI,4, appendix 1) and found again very significant correlations. In general the relationship was closer between two consequtive periods then between distant periods, especially with children. This is understandable as the number of the children and their age varied considerably in the period of observation.

Not only did our investigation of the hundred younger families prove that there were relationships between the frequency of illness in the members of a family, especially between parents and children, but also that the differences between families in frequency of illness tended to be stable over the years. This evidence strongly supports the major thesis that a general practitioner should regard the family as a unit.

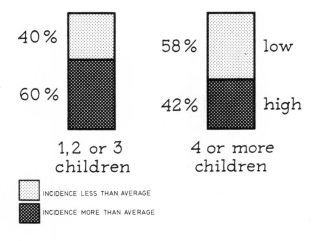

Fig. 9. Incidence of disorders in children and number of children in 100 younger families.

The next step in our investigation was to explore the relationship between the medical data and the psycho-social characteristics of these families, as assessed by the domiciliary team. We wanted to find out how far the differences in frequency of illness, presented to the family doctor, could be explained by these characteristics. We were rather surprised to find that material factors like hygiene, housing and finances (generally supposed to be important), did not prove to be responsible for these differences. The qualities of the mother as a housekeeper and in caring for her children, the social mobility, intelligence and relationship of the father with his children were of doubtful importance. It appeared however that nonmaterial factors like the neurotic stability of the parents, the quality of their marriage relationship and the relationship between the mother and her children were the most important.

To illustrate our findings I will show some diagrams representing the relationship between the incidence of illness in children and some family characteristics. To this end we divided the children of our families into those with more and those with less than the average incidence of disorders. Fig. 9 seems to indicate that in small families more medical help was asked for the children than in large families, as has been found in several other investigations.

This difference however proved not to be statistically important (see table XI,5, appendix 1).
The neurotic stability of the mother (fig. 10) is however of significant importance.(see table XI,6, appendix 1).

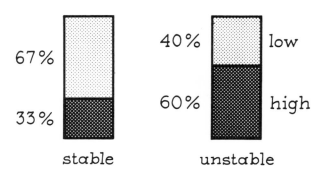

67%

33%

40%   low

60%   high

stable   unstable

Fig. 10. Incidence of disorders and neurotic instability of the mother in 100 younger families.

100

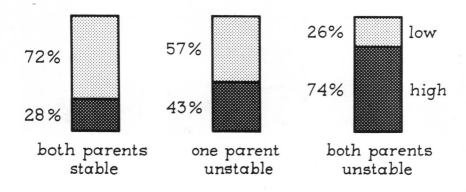

Fig. 11. Incidence of childrens disorders and neurotic instability of both parents in 100 younger families.

Fig. 11 represents the relationship between the stability of both parents and the incidence of disorders in their children. The differences are statistically highly significant (see table XI,7, appendix 1).

Fig. 12 gives a closer look at these differences in different categories of disease. The stability of the parents appeared to have less influence on disorders of the skin and on accidents than on respiratory disorders and nervous disorders of their children (see tables XI, 8-11, appendix 1).

Fig. 13 shows the great importance of the marriage relationship (see table XI, 12, appendix 1). In those families in which the domiciliary team knew there had been problems in this respect, the children were more frequently ill.

It seems probable that disease behaviour (of the parents) is held to be responsible for most of these differences. Nevertheless a family doctor can only combat disease if it is presented to him. Disease behaviour of his patients has far-reaching consequences not only for him, but also for the total health care of the population.

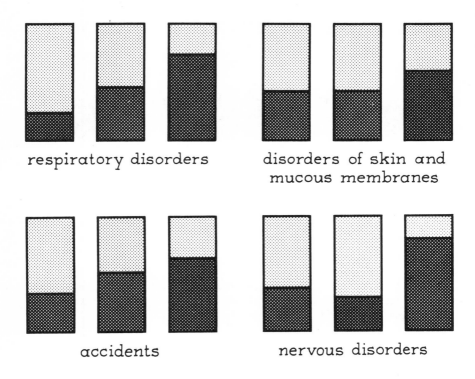

Fig. 12. Incidence of childrens disorders and neurotic instability of both parents in 100 younger families.

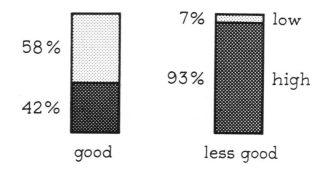

Fig. 13. Incidence of childrens disorders and marriage-relationship of parents in 100 younger families.

XII. A Hundred Older Families

Complementary to the survey of a hundred younger families, described in chapter XI, I later made a similar survey of a hundred older families.
Objectives: the objectives of this study were twofold,
1. to compare the medical data of families in the contracting phase with those of families in the expanding and stabilising phase,
2. to find further evidence to support the thesis demonstrated in younger families that a family doctor must consider the family as a unit of its own.

Methods and material
To this end I collected from my files the records of all couples in the practice who had been married for at least fifteen years at the beginning of the observation-period (1-7-45). The only two criteria for selection were: date of marriage and continuous presence in this practice during the whole observation period (till 1-7-65). Starting with those who married in 1930 I worked backward, adding consecutively all those who married in the earlier years till I had collected the records of one hundred families. Table XII,1 (appendix 1) gives an account of some data of these families.

The comparableness of the younger and older families
The two samples have been taken in a comparable way from the same population. Both the younger and the older families represent all families in a normal general practice. The representation of the social classes is about the same in the samples, higher social classes being under-represented in my practice compared with the population of the whole country.
The medical and social data were collected and coded in the same way, as has been explained in chapter XI, referring to the hundred younger families. The observation period started at the same time (1-7-45), but as the younger couples successively entered the sample by marrying in the years 1946-1948 and as the collection of their data was closed at 1-1-1965, contrasted with 1-7-1965 for the 100 older families, the number of observation years of the younger families is smaller.

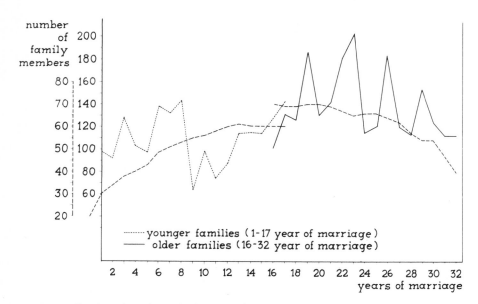

Fig. 14. Total number of consultations per year of marriage of 10 younger + 10 older families.

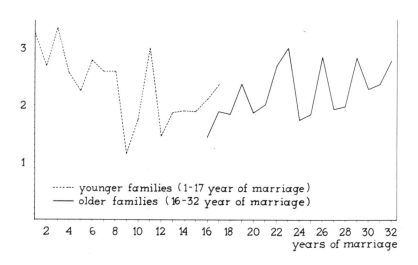

Fig. 15. Average number of consultations per family member per year of marriage, 10 younger + 10 older families.

104

It is evident that the two samples differ in phase of family life as they were selected for this specific purpose. Most of the older families were in the involutionary phase, but still to a few of them children were being born. There are important differences between the two samples inherent to this disparity in family phase, e.g. in the young families parents and children are younger. In the younger families the children entered the observation period as they were born successively, while in the older families they quit the observation period when they left their families. Thus the ratio parents/children is not constant during the span of the observation period: it goes down for the young families and goes up for the older ones. This last effect is partly counteracted by the death of parents. When we add up the numbers for the whole of the observation periods for younger and older families, this difference between younger and older families is more or less counter-balanced. Yet, due to the fact that there were more live-born children in the older (531) than in the younger (378) sample, the relative proportion of children in the total number of patient-years observed is greater in the older families. This will be taken into account when we compare the medical data of the two samples.

A Pilot Study

My partner Van Thiel did a pilot study, comparing the first ten younger and older families. He coded all data himself in exactly the same way. The results of his pilot study are shown in diagrams (fig. 14 to 18) and Table XII,2 (appendix1) gives a summary of some of his figures. There did not appear to be much difference in the general practitioner work load comparing younger and older families, the average number of consultations per family member per year being exactly the same. In the younger families there seemed to have been more emergency consultations and more admissions to hospital. It is self-explanatory that young mothers asked for more maternity care. For illness the older fathers and mothers seemed to have requested more consultations, and the older children less than average.

Looking at the diagram of the total number of consultations of the ten older and ten younger families per year of marriage (fig. 14) we see that the graph goes up for the younger families, with a rather sudden fall in level in the 9th year by which time most of the children had been born. For the older families the graph shows a tendency to fall. However, this variation in the graph of total numbers of consultations cannot be explained precisely by the number of individuals present in the families in the observation period, as is shown in fig. 15, which gives a graph of the average numbers of consultations per family member per year of marriage. This figure suggests a curve with the highest points at the beginning and the end of the observed years of family life and its lowest point in the middle. The left half is explained by fig. 16, presenting the graph of the number of consultations

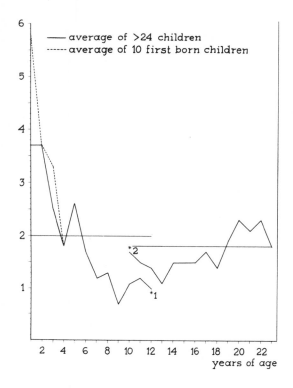

Fig. 16. Total number of consultations per year of age for 10 younger and 10 older families.

* 1 younger families (1-17 year of marriage).
* 2 older families (16-32 year of marriage).

per year of life of the children, showing a steep decline (especially for first born children) while the right half of figure 15 can be explained by the well known fact that ageing people (the parents) consult more.

Of great interest was the breakdown of the different illnesses accounting for the consultations as seen in fig. 17. Infectious diseases, upper respiratory and uro-genital disorders gave rise to fewer consultations in the older families. Figure 18 shows that only nervous disorders caused a continually rising proportion of the consultations over the years of marriage. This seemed to be the most interesting result of this pilot investigation.

The hundred younger and older families
In table XII,3 (appendix 1) some data of the hundred younger and older families are compared. It appears that on the average the older families needed less consultations, that fewer diagnoses were made per year, but the

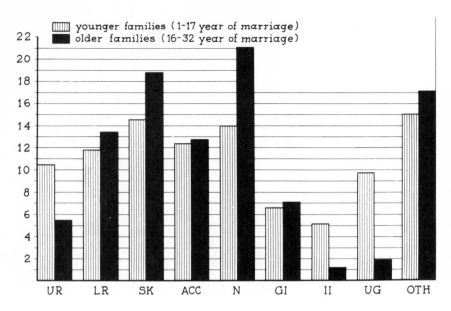

Fig. 17. Percentage of number of consultations per diagnostic category in 10 younger and 10 older families during 17 years.

UR	=	UPPER RESPIRATORY
LR	=	LOWER RESPIRATORY
SK	=	SKIN
ACC	=	ACCIDENTS
N	=	NERVOUS
GI	=	GASTRO-INTESTINAL
II	=	INFECTIOUS DISEASES
UG	=	URO-GENITAL
OTH	=	OTHER

number of consultations per diagnosis went up. This suggests that illnesses lasted longer and/or needed more medical assistance in the older families, as could be expected.

The coded data of consultations and diagnoses are a result of the behaviour of patients and doctor and their interactions. One or both of them could have been different in the two samples. In a retrospective study like this it is not possible to unravel their respective proportions. There are however two sets of rather "hard" data in our material, which provide us with some sort of standard to measure the behaviour of patient and doctor, more or less independently. The emergency or unplanned consultations will practically always have been the result of patient behaviour, while the numbers of referrals and admissions to hospital in most cases will have been a result of doctor behaviour. It is interesting to note that these two

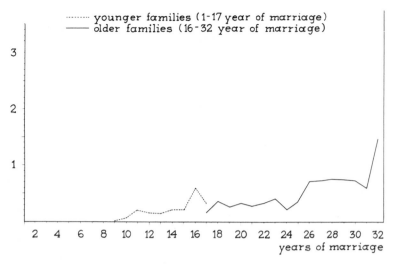

Fig. 18. Number of consultations for nervous disorders per year of marriage for 10 younger and 10 older families.

figures are exactly the same per family member in the younger and older families. This makes it very probable that patient- and doctor behaviour have generally been the same in the two samples. The referral- and admission rates in my practice have always been low in comparison with other Dutch general practitioners.

To compare the *spectrum of morbidity* in the younger and older families we cannot use the method employed in the pilot study, as I could not link the consultations to diagnoses as Van Thiel did. In addition, the number of consultations differ between younger and older families, as do diagnoses. Fig. 19 shows the number of diagnoses in the different illness-categories of the older and the younger families, adjusted to the same number of observation years. In the older families the frequency of disorders appears to have gone down in all disease categories except accidents and nervous disorders, which went up. These changes must be largely due to the children, as these outnumbered the parents by far. In the chapter about the younger families it has been shown indeed that as the children grew up most categories of disease diminished in frequency, the incidence of accidents and nervous disorders alone increased.

Perhaps the changes in the spectrum of morbidity are best demonstrated when we compare the respective percentages of the total number of disorders in the different disease categories, as is done in fig. 20. We see then that in the older families the proportion of upper respiratory, gastro-intestinal, urogenital and other diseases diminished. Infectious diseases almost disappear, the proportions of lower respiratory tract and skin dis-

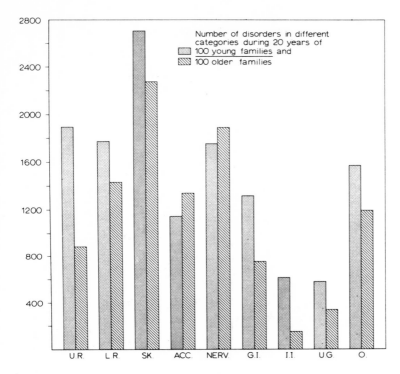

Fig. 19. Number of disorders in different categories during 20 years of 100 younger and 100 older families.

chi-square = 618.568   d.*f.* = 8   p 0,001

UR	=	UPPER RESPIRATORY
LR	=	LOWER RESPIRATORY
SK	=	SKIN
ACC	=	ACCIDENTS
N	=	NERVOUS
GI	=	GASTRO-INTESTINAL
II	=	INFECTIOUS DISEASES
UG	=	URO-GENITAL
OTH	=	OTHER

ease slightly increase, while accidents and nervous disorders occupy a larger share of the spectrum. These changes could be explained by the rise of age in the population. The first objective of this study — the comparison of the medical data of families in the contraction phase with those in the expanding and stabilisation phase — has been achieved with the presentation of these facts.

Objective two of this study was to find further evidence to support the

109

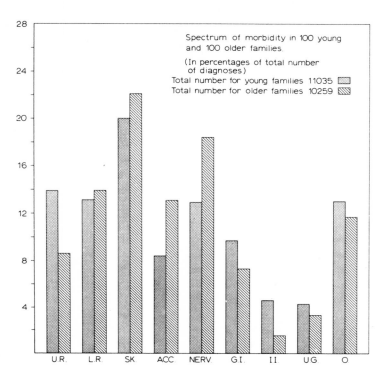

Fig. 20. Spectrum of morbidity in 100 younger and 100 older families. In percentages of total number of diagnoses.

UR	=	UPPER RESPIRATORY
LR	=	LOWER RESPIRATORY
SK	=	SKIN
ACC	=	ACCIDENTS
N	=	NERVOUS
GI	=	GASTRO-INTESTINAL
II	=	INFECTIOUS DISEASES
UG	=	URO-GENITAL
OTH	=	OTHER

thesis that a family doctor must regard the family as an unit of its own. In looking for this evidence we have two different kinds of data to work with: medical and social. In the medical data perhaps a distinction can be made between the predominantly patient-induced data, such as consultations and emergency consultations on the one hand, and predominantly doctor-induced data like diagnoses, referrals and admissions to hospital on the other hand. In reality these last two categories of data are interrelated, it being impossible for instance for the doctor to make a diagnosis without a consultation by the patient.

Method

All medical data was computed to figures per patient-year for father, mother and "family-child". Patient-year was defined as the average of all years the patient stayed in his family during the observation period, irrespective of the fact whether the doctor had seen him or not. "Family-child" was defined as the average of all children in the sample belonging to the same family, scaled to one child to standardize the family size.

As a result the families in this part of the study were reduced to a composite family of father, mother and one "family-child". Further details of method will be given with the results.

Results

1. *Diagnoses*

In the 89 familes with children we examined the relationship between fathers, mothers and children regarding the total number of their diagnoses (see table XII,4 appendix 1). As with the younger families we found a statistically very significant similarity. This means that if one of the parents had many periods of illness it was likely not only that the children but also the other parent would show the same phenomenon.

The correlations between parents and children were much greater than that between the parents themselves. In the younger families the correlation was highest between mother and children, in the older families the correlation between father and children was even higher.

It can be concluded that considering the total number of diagnoses (= periods of illness) we have again found evidence of consistency within the family unit.

After the total number of periods of illness we looked at the number of diagnoses in the various categories of disease used in this study (see table XII,5, appendix 1). The prevalence of disorders of the skin, of the lower respiratory tract and (to a somewhat lesser degree) of gastro-intestinal and nervous disorders, and of accidents proved to be familial. (In nervous disorders the correlations were only significant between father and mother, while there were no significant correlations between the parents for accidents and gastro-intestinal disorders).

For the disease categories, which showed significant "familiarity" a family index was computed and a correlation matrix was made, which was factor analysed (see table XII,6, appendix 1). The frequency of illness in all these categories proved to be highly significantly interrelated and only one factor came out. This to me was a rather unexpected result, as I had thought it possible that some families were especially prone to accidents, others to nervous disorders or to lower respiratory tract — or skin diseases. But it proved that the vulnerability of the families was evenly spread over the different disease categories. Another explanation could be that the common factor has to be looked for in the general illness-behaviour of the families. If this last explanation is correct it could be predicted that the consultation indices of the family members will show high correlation.

2. *Consultations*

For the normal consultations, emergency consultations, referrals to specialists and admissions to hospital, an index was constructed for the whole 20 year observation period for fathers, mothers and children, in the same way as explained for diagnoses. We again looked for similarities between the family members (see table XII,7, appendix 1), but it transpired that only with referrals could one demonstrate some familial similarity. This considerably differs from the same figures for diagnoses, making it less probable in my opinion that illness behaviour has to be regarded as the explanation in the familial character of disease, as described in the preceding paragraphs.

The social data

A family index was constructed (see table XII,8 and 9, appendix 1) for each of the activities (normal consultations, emergency consultations, referrals and admissions to hospital). We investigated the relationships between these indices of (doctor induced) diagnoses and (patient induced) consultations with several measurements of social data. To achieve this we used the year of marriage, the number of viable children, the families' social class and the scores derived from four factors obtained from factor-analysis of psycho-social data, described in chapter XI concerning the younger families.

These factors were believed to be 1) influence of father, 2) influence of mother, 3) psycho-social burden of the family and 4) material situation of the family.

The results of this investigation are in table XII,10 (appendix 1). It appeared that families of the higher social classes tended to have had less disorders and to have asked for less consultations, while large families tended to have had less consultations per family member per year. This last finding is in accord with the results of the younger families survey. Families with a heavier social burden tended to have had more consultations per family member. This part of our investigation did not surprise us with important unexpected results.

Finally we examined in detail the relationship between the numbers of diagnoses and consultations for fathers, mothers and children in each family, as it seemed to us these interactions within the family were important in family medicine (see table XII,11, appendix 1). Again highly significantly positive correlations between the numbers of diagnoses of parents and children, and a significant, but less strong positive correlation between father and mother came to light. On the other hand, there were no significant correlations between the consultation indices of the family members. The total number of diagnoses appeared to be connected with the total number of consultations for the parents but not for the children. The number of contacts with the parents proved to be connected with the number of diagnoses in their children, but the consultation index of the children did not show any significant correlation with other indices.

Summing up the findings of this chapter on the hundred older families we have evidence that the spectrum of morbidity, seen by the family doctor, proved indeed to be different from that of the younger families. Some categories such as upper-respiratory disease and infectious disease decreased in importance, while accidents and nervous disorders needed more medical attention. It seems most probable that these changes can be explained by the age differences.

The results of statistical analysis again supported my main thesis in this book that a general practitioner needs to consider the family as a unit. The consistency within the family proved however to be far more important for the total numbers of diagnoses than for the total numbers of consultations. Examining different kinds of disease, evidence was found to suppose one common factor responsible for this consistency within the family, or "familiarity" of illness. A common illness-behaviour of the family could be this factor, but this was less probable by finding that this consistency within the families was absent for their total numbers of consultations. I suggest this factor is called the *vulnerability* of the family. It may be important for the family doctor to realize that families not only differ in their readiness to call his help (which he will know from experience), but perhaps also in their readiness to fall a prey to all kinds of disease.

XIII. A Comparison of the 100 family studies with morbidity data of later years

Some time ago one of my staff members told me how he had been working as a doctor in a developing country for some years. It had been a great satisfaction for him to be able to observe that in a short time several diseases disappeared and that the health of the population improved visibly. His story had an unexpected effect on me, I caught myself being jealous. The wish to cure people and to make them more healthy had been my most important motive to study medicine. Suddenly I realized that the health of the population for which I had been working day and night for more than thirty years seemed only to have deteriorated and I felt depressed.

Indeed, statistics of the Netherlands show that the mortality per 1000 inhabitants has gone up in the last 30 years and the percentage of sickness absenteeism has duplicated. Of the working population, 10% is now thought to be permanently disabled.

The data of the 100 families analysed in chapter XI and XII enabled me to make an estimation of the frequency of illness for which medical help was called in between 1945 and 1975 by the population I have been serving as family doctor. Figures 21 and 22 give the numbers of all disorders presented to me by the old and young families in 1946-1965 and of the whole practice population in 1971-1975 computed per 1000 per year according to age and sex. These data comprise almost 50.000 observed patient-years. The way of analysis and presentation is such that in the data of the old families the years of observation of 1945-1955 predominate and in the data of the young families the years of observation of 1955-1965. The figures make clear that for both males and females in practically each of the age categories examined the number of disorders presented to the family doctor increases from old via young families to the level of the last years. The graphs show that all age and sex categories in my practice presented in 1971-1975 almost twice as many disorders to the doctor as did the members of the old families 20 to 30 years ago.

Can these striking differences be attributed to changes in my way of making diagnoses? It seems likely that I have become more acute in diagnosing disorders such as obesity and hypertension, but I think it

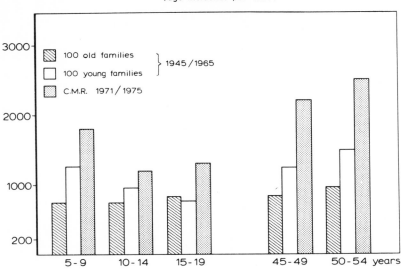

Fig. 21.

total number of disorders in men
(age incidence per 1000)

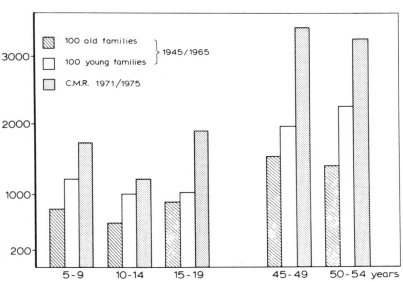

total number of disorders in women
Fig. 22. (age incidence per 1000)

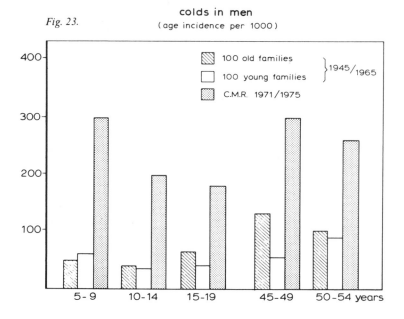

Fig. 23.

colds in men
(age incidence per 1000)

100 old families
100 young families   } 1945/1965
C.M.R. 1971/1975

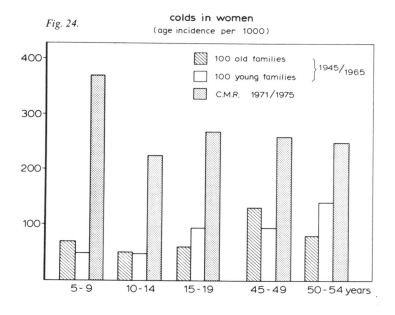

Fig. 24.

colds in women
(age incidence per 1000)

100 old families
100 young families   } 1945/1965
C.M.R. 1971/1975

116

improbable that this can explain the large and systematic differences observed in all kinds of disorders. Further analysis revealed that the kind of disorder or disease had influence on these differences. Figures 23 and 24 show that in colds there were minor differences between old and young families, but enormous differences between then and nowadays, especially for young children. Infectious skin diseases (figure 25 and 26) have diminished in frequency, perhaps due to better hygiene.

Age and sex also appeared to have influence. Figures 27 and 28 show that nervous disorders hardly increased in children (especially in boys). Mothers of young families had more nervous symptoms than mothers of old families and women of these age categories in the last years, while the numbers of nervous symptoms of men in the last years exceed those of the fathers of the young and old families. Perhaps this reflects a diminishing stress on women and an increasing stress on men.

Nervous disorders and colds are rather "soft" diagnoses, liable to subjective factors in doctor and patient. But a much more "hard" diagnosis such as otitis media (always made by examination of the eardrums) also shows interesting trends (figures 29 and 30): striking increase in young children, hardly any difference in the 10-14 age categories.

Urinary tract infection, a diagnosis which was always based on microscopical investigation, appears to have increased in women of all age categories examined (see figure 31).

These figures raise several interesting questions such as: has the incidence of colds and otitis in children really risen or do parents call the doctor more readily nowadays? Do I look more often at the eardrums of children with a cold and do I examine the urine of women more frequently? As far as I know my practice routine has not changed considerably. I do not think that this can be the explanation of the differences observed. Besides this, it can be said that the opinion of general practitioners in my country as a whole points in the same direction: all of them with long standing experience agree that they are more often consulted for health disturbances by their practice population then they used to be. If we define illness as a deviation of health for which medical help is called in, there can be little doubt that there is a substantial increase of illness in the population in the last thirty years. There can also be little doubt that in defining illness in this way the medical profession and health care in general have played an active role in this increase of unhealthiness.

Supply increases demand, also in the medical field. By offering my services continuously during the past thirty years I have maintained and stimulated the increased medical demands in my practice. Now I find myself in the paradoxical situation in which one of my most important tasks is to protect my patients from undue medical interference and its ensuing inherent dangers. These dangers are most imminent when people are referred to specialists. Then many unnecessary investigations and ad-

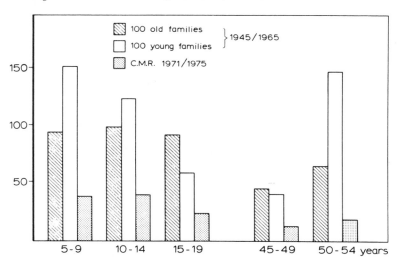

Fig. 25.

infections of skin in men

(age incidence per 1000)

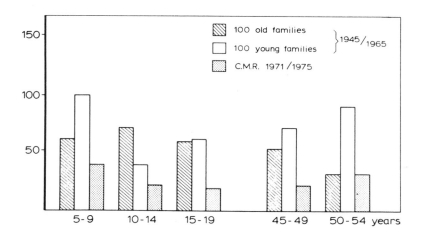

Fig. 26.

infections of skin in women

(age incidence per 1000)

118

nervous disorders in men

Fig. 27.

(age incidence per 1000)

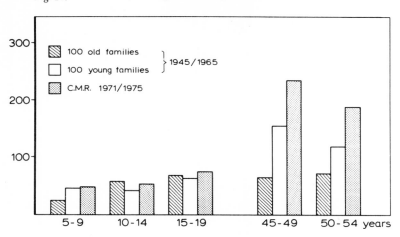

nervous disorders in women

Fig. 28.

(age incidence per 1000)

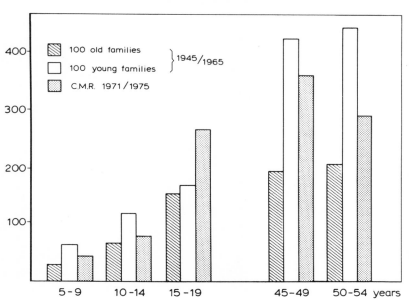

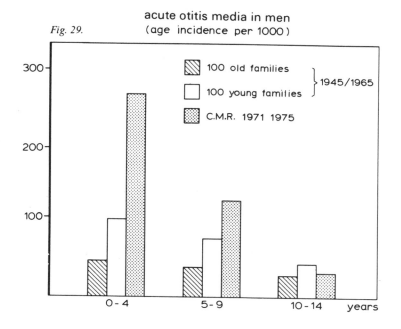

Fig. 29.

acute otitis media in men
(age incidence per 1000)

100 old families
100 young families } 1945/1965
C.M.R. 1971 1975

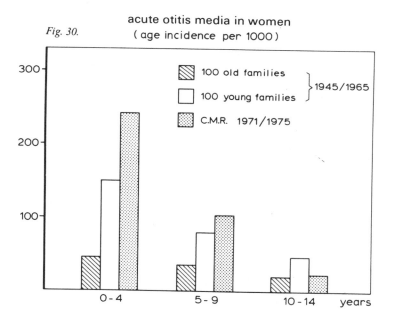

Fig. 30.

acute otitis media in women
(age incidence per 1000)

100 old families
100 young families } 1945/1965
C.M.R. 1971/1975

120

missions to hospital, all done more to exclude than to discover serious disease, will be inevitable. Minor deviations from hypothetical "norms" and even physiological variations are apt to be regarded as "pathological" and to be treated as such, making healthy people patients, dependent upon health professionals. In my practice the hospital admission rate is only half the average of the country and still I suspect that about half the number of days my patients spend in hospital are not strictly indicated (i.e. no procedures are undertaken which are indicated and for which hospitalisation of the patient is indispensable). The investigations and treatments they are subjected to are by no means always harmless, sometimes even making them really ill. In this way people are caught in vicious circles from which they cannot escape by themselves. An inclination to perfectionism and a fear to make omissions or failures on the part of the specialist can lead to serious iatrogenic harm in the patient. I have seen many examples of this in my practice. Often the reasons for patients entering these medical labyrinths should be sought in the psycho-social sphere or in their families. But in the course of events these causes fade away into the background and become inaccessable. It is almost impossible for a general practitioner to prevent this once his patients are referred to specialists. More and more referrals for purely diagnostic reasons are regarded by specialists as a reason to take over the whole treatment automatically and indefinitely. In my opinion it would be far better if specialists acted more like consultants as they did in former days, advising the general practitioner and only taking over the treatment if and when this is strictly necessary.

It is a pity that the medical schools where specialists are trained give bad examples in this respect. Evidently changes to the better will only be possible if general practitioners will be competent physicians with a thorough training and with keen medical interests, combining this with psychological and social sensitivities and abilities. They should only refer what they cannot do themselves and even then try to keep contact with their patients in order to be able to guide them. As a generalist the family doctor has a better over-all view of the whole person in his social context. Naturally the specialist is bothered in the first place with specific medical problems and he is not in the best position to judge the whole person and the interactions in the family system.

The general practitioner will have to be able to weigh critically the pro's and con's of different kinds of treatment and interventions in order to advise his patients. Above all however he will have to try to place and keep the responsibility for actions where this belongs, with the patient himself and with his family. The independence and self-care of people must be furthered whereever possible.

People are expecting far too much from medical care nowadays. They think that medicine can take away from them almost all kinds of disease and discomfort, if medical advice is only called in betimes. In reality, the

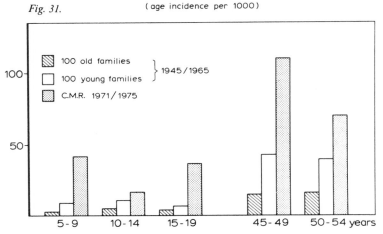

Fig. 31.

acute urinary infections in women
(age incidence per 1000)

power of medicine to heal and to cure is very limited indeed. The book on the role of medicine in the last three centuries in England and Wales written by Thomas McKeown (1976) and other critical studies make this abundantly clear. We doctors have been fooling both ourselves and the population and it is time we stop doing so and learn to be realistic. But since these unrealistic expectations have reached such gigantic proportions it will be very difficult for us to fight them. There is even reason to believe that similar unrealistic expectations are now being stimulated by psychotherapists and social scientists.

The old adage describing the tasks of the practising doctor as "to cure sometimes, to relieve often, to comfort always" is still true. I would only prefer to replace the word "comfort" with "helping to live with illness and disability". This wish to be comforted, to be relieved and, if possible, to be cured by the doctor seems however to have spread and grown in the population. I have little doubt that the family plays an important role in the spreading of these expectations.

Reference:
McKeown, Thomas (1976), The role of medicine. Dream, mirage, or nemesis? The Nuffield Provincial Hospital Trust.

XIV. A Three-Generation Family Study

Introduction

In 1970 Heijdendael, a psychologist, Mrs. Ketelaar-van Ierssel and Persoon, sociologists, and myself as a general practitioner, collaborated on an intensive exploratory investigation into a sample of three generations families. The details were published in a book we wrote about this study (Heijdendael e.a. 1972). In this chapter I will review only our major conclusions for two reasons. The first reason is that some of the findings described in the earlier chapters were confirmed, while others were not, proving things to be more complicated then we anticipated and perhaps I should tell my readers about this.

The second reason is that our exploratory investigation might give others a starting point for further research.

Objects of study

The main objects of our combined three-generation study were to specify and analyse psychological, sociological and medical family data and to explore the correlations between these facts. This chapter is limited mostly to correlations between the psycho-social and medical data.

Material and methods

Our sample comprised about a hundred families composed of three generations. The oldest and the middle-aged families were chosen at random from the "older" and "younger" families, described in chapter XI and XII of this book. We did this to be able to investigate their psycho-social characteristics in more depth. The youngest families were chosen at random from the family-register of my practice, the only criterion being that their year of marriage had to be around 1960. The youngest families therefore had been married about 10 years, the middle families about 25 years and the oldest about 40 years at the time of our study. All of these families have been visited by five medical students who had been trained in interviewing techniques. The fathers and the mothers in all families and one of the oldest children in the middle and old families were interviewed with standard questions. They had to fill in their questionnaires separately, but simultaneously, without discussion or collaboration. Table XIV,1 (appendix 1) gives the numbers of the children and the social classes of these families.

The medical data of the years 1967, 1968 and 1969, not included in the previous studies, were used now, diagnoses having been coded according to the Royal College of General Practitioners "E" book list since 1-1-1967 for the whole practice. The diagnoses were grouped into the same categories as used in the hundred younger and older families, adding an additional category for preventive actions. Numbers of consultations, referrals to specialists and admissions to hospital were counted per individual per year. The psycho-social data can be divided into the predominantly individual and predominantly inter-individual data. The individual data we collected included an intelligence screening test (Kent Series of Emergency Scales), a test of neurotic instability (Amsterdamse Biographische Vragenlijst, a questionnaire similar to the Eysenck personality inventory) and a list of items concerning the individual's concept of "the good father", "the good mother" and "the good child".

The inter-individual data collected can be subdivided into those concerning the parental relationship and those concerning the parent-child relationship. We investigated the parent-child relationship, both from the parents' viewpoint as well as from the child's. We used for the parent-child relationship the Schaefer Parental Attitude Research Instrument (both father-child and mother-child), and for the child-parent relationship the Parental Behaviour Research Instrument (also designed by Schaefer and divided into child-father and child-mother). Parents were not only questioned as to their attitudes towards their children, but also regarding their childhood experience of their own fathers' and mothers' behaviour.

Assessing the marriage relationship we used many questions from the Dutch Statistical Society's marriage questionnaire, creating a new method to determine the degree of discordancy between the partners over their behaviour, their ideas and their wishes spanning several aspects of life. Not only did we ask husband and wife what they thought about these aspects, but also how they anticipated their partners would answer. In this way we could score both real and perceived discrepancy, problem areas in marriage and mutual degrees of satisfaction of husband and wife with their daily work and life.

Results

The medical data showed a marked consistency during the three years of the period of observation. This was demonstrable for the total numbers of disorders (diagnoses), the numbers of diagnoses in several categories and for the total numbers of consultations, referrals and admissions to hospital. This was not only true for fathers, mothers and children separately, but also

124

for families as a whole. This consistency could not be attributed to chronic illnesses.

The hypotheses postulated in the earlier chapters, that in illness the family has to be regarded as a unit, and that families tend to be consistent in illness patterns over the years, were amply confirmed. Again it was demonstrated that the factor (or several factors) responsible for this consistency must have influenced all disease categories.

On analysing the medical data, close agreement was found between numbers of illnesses and of consultations, but less agreement between these and referrals and admissions. This makes it less probable that the general practitioner could have been an important agent to explain the consistency demonstrated. The striking fact, that little correlation was found between nervous symptoms and others, which was later confirmed in a more extensive investigation covering three other large general practices, contradicted the popular belief that individuals and families with nervous symptoms tend to call on the doctor more often also for other illness.

An endeavour to construct a family typology, based on categories of disease, failed. Increase in frequency of illnesses went with diminishing specificity of disease categories. Further research is needed to clarify the differences of medical "vulnerability" between families.

The *family-phase* showed high correlation with several aspects of the medical data. As families aged, more fathers had more illnesses and consultations, while mothers of young and middle families had more illnesses and consultations than mothers in old families. This suggested that the strain on fathers increased with years, but decreased in mothers of old families. The children of young families showed the most diseases and consultations, children of middle families the least. Generally the medical data confirmed the results of the 100 younger and older families study.

Contrary to expectation, the number of diseases and consultations of both parents and their children appeared to be independant of the *neurotic instability* and *intelligence* of the parents. This is in contradition not only with the findings of Hare and Shaw (1965), Kellner (1963), Buck and Laughton (1959) and other investigators, but also with data in chapter XI about the hundred younger families. It was also disquieting to find that the correlations were low between the domiciliary team's estimation of the parent's neurotic instability and the questionnaires for neurosis (The Amsterdam Biographische Vragenlijst), especially for fathers. This A.B.V. is meant to measure he neurotic instability as a constant behaviour characteristic of personality, not as a measure of present potentially variable neurotic symptoms. It is possible that the members of the domiciliary team allowed their judgement of personality characteristics to be influenced by present symptoms. It is also possible that the A.B.V. does not measure what it purports. The fact that there were practically no significant positive correlations between A.B.V. score and either numbers of nervous symptoms, or total number of diseases and consultations, seems to make its use by general practitioners of doubtful valu. The A.B.V. and similar devices used often by psychologists to attempt to measure neurotic instability instrumently will have to be validated in general practice.

The *social-economic class* of the father appears to show definite correlations with his total number of illnesses and consultations, while the *number of children* showed significant but negative correlations with their (and their mother's) medical data. This confirms the finding of both the hundred family studies in previous chapters and also those of Brenkman (1963), Hare and Shaw (1965) and Picken and Ireland (1969). It may be that in large families there is relatively less attention for each child and perhaps also for the mother who cannot allow herself to become ill, but it could also be argued that large families indeed promote health by providing healthy stimuli and many challenges. Some of the most intriguing results of our three-generation family study concerned the *relationships between parents and children*. There proved to be hardly any significant correlation between the educational attitudes and expectations of the parents as stated by themselves, and the practical experience of the children from their parents actual behaviour in reality. The same fascinating discrepancy applied to the relationships between the parents' childhood experiences and their present educational attitudes. Either Schaefer's instruments used are no good or these relations in real life are seldom as straight-forward as assumed by most psychologists in their daily professional transactions with patients!

Between fathers and mothers of the same family there also existed very significant differences between the actual experience and the interpretation of the educational situation. Anyhow we were forced to draw the conclusion, most important for the daily practice of family doctors and all others who have to deal professionally with families, that one has to be very cautious indeed in assuming that information about the family given by one member agrees with the real truth.

Again, contrary to our expectations, in this survey the father's educational attitude seemed to have more influence upon the medical consultations and illnesses of the children during their upbringing than the mother's. A relationship between the children's experience of their mother's behaviour and their own medical demands, appeared only in a later period of their lives. Childrens' experiences of their mother's behaviour in this respect seemed to have more and further reaching consequences.

Progressive or traditional thinking about their own *role*, or the child's role in the family, hardly appeared to make a difference in the consultations for illness of parents and children. It struck us that in this population the parents thought far more conservatively about the child's role than about their own roles. For future research it seems desirable to investigate in depth the concept and impact of role-insecurity.

The *marriage relationship* variables, especially disagreement between partners, showed numerous correlations with the medical data of the partners and their children. This emphasized an important source of trouble in the medical field, confirming the findings in chapter XI of this book dealing with the 100 younger families. Disagreement between the parents had more repercussions on the medical data of their children (especially in old families) than on their own medical data. Astonishing differences became apparent between real and supposed subjects of discord between the parents with real discord observed least in the older couples.

In each of the aspects of the marriage relationship examined however, the percentage of husbands and wives who confessed to problems was lower than observed. The major concealed problem was sex. Both husbands and wives named the children's education as their first most important problem and financial worries as the second. Women listed sexual and religious problems more often than men. Questioned about whom they consulted for their marriage problems (either professionals or non-profesionals), both husbands and wives named the general practitioner first.

In the inter-correlation of the psycho-social data, clear agreement became apparent between neurotic instability (especially of men) and marriage problems. Both identifying the problems and seeking advice in this field varied chiefly with neurotic instability.

Our inter-disciplinary investigation was of an exploratory nature, and our findings cannot as such be extrapolated to other populations for whom further research will be necessary. Our investigation was not really longitudinal: we compared different families who started their family life in different times. Real on-going longitudinal family research data would be invaluable. The general practitioner has inherent opportunities to investigate this if he has the advantage that families stay with him for years. In our project we tried to focus on the family as the unit of investigation and this proved fruitful, but the relationships within the family were revealed to be very complex. We suggest that further research should aim not only at individual and isolated aspects, but should give priority to inter-individual variables such as the intra-familial relationships and the relationships between the family and the outer world, including norms and cultural orientations. Attitudes and behaviour to health, disease and health care deserve far more attention than they have hitherto recieved.

References:

Brenkman, C.F. (1963), De huisarts en het gezin van zijn patiënt, Assen.

Buck, C.W. and K.B. Laughton (1959), Family patterns of illness. The effect of psychoneurosis in the parent upon illness in the child. Acta Psych. Neurolog. Scandin. 34, 165.

Hare, E.H. and G.K. Shaw (1965), A study in family health: health in relation to family size. Brit. J. psych., 111, 461 en 467.

Heydendael, P.H.J.M. e.a. (1972), Gezin en Ziekte, Dekker & van de Vegt, Nijmegen.

Kellner, R. (1963), Family illness. An investigation in general practice. London.

Picken, P. and G. Ireland (1969), Family-patterns of medical care utilization. Possible influences of family-size, role and social class on illness-behaviour. J. chron. diseases, 22, 181.

Schaefer, E.S. (1957), Organization of maternal behavior and attitudes within a two-dimensional space: an application of Guttman's Radex Theory. The Am. psychol., 12, 401.

Schaefer, E.S. (1959), A circumplex model for maternal behavior. J. abn. soc. psychol., 59, 226.

Schaefer, E.S. (1961), Converging conceptual models for maternal behavior and for child behavior. In: Parental attitudes and child behavior, ed. by J. Glidewell, Springfield.

Schaefer, E.S. and R.Q. Bell (1957), Patterns of attitudes toward child rearing and the family. J. abn. soc. psychol., 54, 381.

Schaefer, E.S. (1958), Development of a parental research instrument. Child developm., 29, 338.

128

XV. Further Family Investigations

When I was appointed to the Medical Faculty of Nijmegen University to teach what was called "the application of medicine in the family" and started the University Institute of General Practice, I became involved in teaching and organizing, and had little time for investigation. I then had a sociologist and a psychologist on my staff and together we decided to undertake a further exploration of medical family life with the help of students. The analysis of the data is not finished yet and I will only mention some of the most important results here.

I. A Study of 200 Families

Object of study. We knew by then of the familiality of illness as presented to the doctor, and we wondered how this phenomenon was to be explained. The object of this study was to find out factors which could be brought into relation with this familiality.

Material and methods. In 1970 210 complete families (father and mother and at least 1 child at home) were chosen at random from my practice file. The children had to be 12-22 years old, the parents' ages ranged from 40 to 64. Families which had participated in the study of chapter XIV were excluded. Each family was visited three times by medical students, who collected the following data of parents and children separately:

— their general *sense of well-being*
— the *kind and number of symptoms* experienced in the last fortnight and what they had done about these (three times)
— their *medical knowledge* by filling out a simple test of 25 questions
— their *anxiety* by making use of an abbreviated version of Taylor's "Manifest Anxiety Scale"
— their *confrontation* with serious illness or death in their neighbourhood
— their *readiness to seek medical help* by confronting them with 27 hypothetical illness situations and asking them what they would do in these circumstances.

All this data was related to the numbers of diagnoses recorded by the general practitioner in the computer file of continuous morbidity registration and to the number of contacts with the g.p. in 1967-1970.

Results

On computation there appeared to be highly significant correlations between the family members in their general sense of wellbeing and in their number of symptoms experienced. This number of symptoms proved to differ markedly from individual to individual, but tended to be stable for each individual, also for symptoms for which no medical help had been sought (about 90% of all symptoms). The most important results regarding the interrelations between the family members are presented in table 15.1.

It is not surprising that the concordance between the parents is highest for confrontation with serious illness. Between father and children this concordance coefficient is twice as high as between mother and children, indicating that the father seems to be the most important mediator. In medical knowledge there is also a high agreement between the parents and somewhat less between parents and children, with no difference between father and mother. Anxiety proved to be hardly familial, only the concordance between mother and children being significant. In readiness to seek medical help and in the number of contacts with the g.p. significant familiality could be established. The most striking result of this investigation in my opinion was however that this familiality was far more

Table 15.1. *Concordance within the family, between parents and between both parents and their children.*

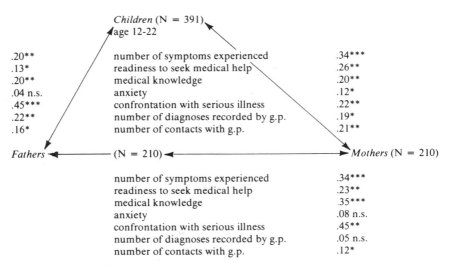

	Children (N = 391) age 12-22	
.20**	number of symptoms experienced	.34***
.13*	readiness to seek medical help	.26**
.20**	medical knowledge	.20**
.04 n.s.	anxiety	.12*
.45***	confrontation with serious illness	.22**
.22**	number of diagnoses recorded by g.p.	.19*
.16*	number of contacts with g.p.	.21**

Fathers ◄——— (N = 210) ◄——————————► Mothers (N = 210)

	number of symptoms experienced	.34***
	readiness to seek medical help	.23**
	medical knowledge	.35***
	anxiety	.08 n.s.
	confrontation with serious illness	.45**
	number of diagnoses recorded by g.p.	.05 n.s.
	number of contacts with g.p.	.12*

n.s.	=	not significant
*	=	significant (p < .05)
**	=	very significant (p < .01)
***	=	highly significant (p < .001)

130

outspoken in the number of symptoms experienced, for which (in more then 90%) no medical help was sought. This finding makes it highly improbable that the familiality of illness as presented to the doctor can be explained simply by a common disease-behaviour within the family. A common liability to symptoms of ill-health seems to be of more importance.

II. *An Extensive and Intensive Family Study*
Gradually my department enlarged. Since 1970 three other general practices are participating in our computer based continuous morbidity registration: one in a village, the second one in a small town and a third one in a big city. The investigations I have been describing in this book all took place in my own practice. The question rose as to whether these results could be confirmed by investigations in a broader field. To this end we analysed the morbidity presented to the general practitioner in 1973-1976 in all four practices linked to our Institute, looking especially at the relationships in numbers of diagnoses between parents and children. Fig. 32 based on the data of a population of more than 3300 children, makes it abundantly clear that they presented least illness when both their parents needed the doctor less than average, that the number of diagnoses rose when their father, and still more when their mother needed the doctor often, while the number of diagnoses of the children was highest when both parents needed the doctor more than average. So we can conclude that the relationship between the frequency of illness of parents and children is not limited to my practice.

Fig. 32. Scores of recorded morbidity of 3332 children in relationship to recorded morbidity of their parents.

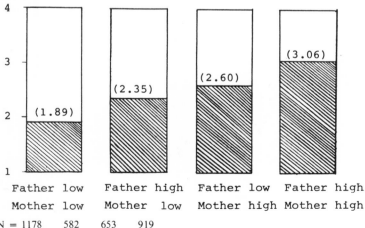

N = 1178   582   653   919
SCORE 1 = children with least morbidity (first quartile)
SCORE 4 = children with highest morbidity (last quartile).

131

The psychologists and sociologists of my department took a stratified sample of 405 families from the four practices, after having divided all families into three groups: those with low, with high and with intermediate registered morbidity. They did an intensive investigation of these families, this time with the help of trained sociological interviewers. The *object* of this study was to find family characteristics which could be brought into relation with the differences in the presentation of illness. The details of methods and results in this investigation will be published elsewhere, but it seems appropriate to tell the readers of this book that we were indeed able to find relevant factors. Perhaps the most important finding is that the relevant psycho-social characteristics of the parents showed a stronger relationship with the frequency of illness of their children than with their own. This offers possibilities for prevention, in trying to disrupt the chain of events in handing down illness from generation to generation as described earlier in this book.

Table 15.2 shows the most relevant relationships between the psycho-social characteristics of the parents and the number of diagnoses of the children, recorded by the general practitioners.

Table 15.2 Relationship between recorded morbidity of 700 children and psycho-social characteristics of their parents

	Kendall's tau coefficient
Tendency to avoid conflicts of father	.09**
Tendency to avoid conflicts of mother	.16***
Flexibility of parental relationship	.01
Involvement in social networks of father	.01
Involvement in social networks of mother	−.13***
Proneness to bodily complaints of father	.06*
Proneness to bodily complaints of mother	.12**
Subjective health of father	−.08**
Subjective health of mother	−.06*
Inclination to accept sick role by father	−.04
Inclination to accept sick role by mother	.05(*)
Readiness to seek medical help by father	−.04
Readiness to seek medical help by mother	−.01
Discrepancy between parents in knowledge with complaints of partner	.09**

(*) $.05 <$ $p < .10$
* $p < .05$
** $p < .01$
*** $p < .001$

It can be seen that children needed the doctor more often when:
— their parents tended to avoid conflicts
— their mother was little involved in social networks outside the family

132

- their parents were prone to somatic complaints
- their parents had a less than average sense of general wellbeing
- their mother was strongly inclined to accept the sick-role
- there was a discrepancy in their parents' knowledge of complaints of the partner.

It is worthy to note that there was no relationship demonstrable in the inclination of the parents to seek medical aid when confronted with (hypothetical) health problems.

All this seems to point in the direction of the projection mechanism described by Balint (1956) as "the child as a presenting symptom". Failure to cope with internal conflicts and with health problems of the parents seems to result in presenting illness of the children to the doctor. Further analysis of our data brought to light that these psycho-social characteristics of the parents hardly played a role in this respect if they themselves already often visited the doctor. This can be interpreted as additional evidence for the existence of projection mechanisms within the family.

This investigation confirmed that (the presentation of) illness has to do with the way people communicate and interact within the family unit.

As a consequence we are working out new experimental measures to prevent what we call "somatic fixation" in families. We are trying to develop instruments for general practitioners to spot in time families liable to these mechanisms. We will try to sensitize g.p.'s and offer them and these families possibilities of programs aimed at prevention of canalisations of internal conflicts in somatic complaints, ending up in inappropiate medical channels, with inherent dangers of confirming unsound behaviour and iatrogenic harm.

Reference:
Balint, M. (1956), The Doctor, His Patient and The Illness, Pitman Medical Publishing Co, London.

XVI. Family Therapy

Introduction

Family therapy is mostly done by psychotherapists. General practitioners do not seem to have much experience with this kind of therapy in which the family unit is the patient. I know of only a few publications about family therapy from general practice, those of Tomm (1973) and Comley (1973). In this chapter I will describe our experiences with family therapy in the department of general practice of the Nijmegen University.

Why we started

Several reasons can be given for starting with this kind of therapy. To start with a negative argument, it can be stated that the effects of the usual kind of psychotherapy are disappointing and almost negligible compared to the enormous amount of psychosocial problems with which a general practitioner is confronted in his daily life. The conventional psychotherapy is individual-centered and directed at intraindividual processes while every general practitioner will know from experience that in reality his patients usually get bogged down in the problem of relating to others. Several case studies in this book illustrate that these relationship problems are passed on in families from generation to generation. Family therapy offers the possibility to break and modify this chain of events as it is not primarily directed at individuals but at their mutual relationships. Individual physical illness can only explain a minor part of the variance in the appeal made to a general practitioner by his patients. Illness behaviour is much more important in this respect. To behave like a patient and to call on a doctor is to a large extent usually a sequence of human interactions in the living and working systems in society. In the family system children learn to behave and they also learn illness behaviour. Family therapy opens up the perspective of prevention. Besides this it can be said that behaving like a patient not only has causes but also consequences especially in the family and often it has more or less (sub)-conscious meanings. It is especially toward these mechanisms that family therapy is directed.

What we did

The readers of this book will not be surprised to learn that the philosophy of family therapy appealed to me when we came into connection with the branch of family therapy of the Nijmegen School of Social Work. Two of our psychologists completed a training in family therapy and our department started a systematic collaboration with the department of family therapy in which we supplied the families they needed for their trainees. In combined meetings the staff of both departments structured this collaboration and laid down rules. We designed forms for request, report and follow up, enabling us to evaluate what was going on. All in all, up till now some 300 families were taken in therapy. Most of these families belonged to practices of general practitioners, staff members of my institute. I will try to give an idea of what we learned.

Two case histories

For us, general practitioners, the collaboration with the family therapists was an experience which differed greatly from what we were accustomed to in referring patients to psychiatrists. Perhaps I can best try to illustrate this with two case histories.

Mrs. Poppy was a trim and very polite woman, a model housewife for her husband and four children.She had always been a bit anxious but recently she had become depressed and was bothered by thoughts of suicide. Again and again she became panic-stricken and called in the help of neighbours, relatives, the priest and others. During the past few years eight professional helpers had tried to relieve her, without much success. Sometimes the helpers, like our social case worker who specialized in crisis intervention, had taken considerable pains, but all was in vain. She got worse and worse. Her husband often phoned me about her and he himself started to complain about fears of having a coronary infarction. The eldest son suffered inceasingly from migraine headaches and the youngest started to wet his bed again. The eldest daughter also began to have anxieties and feared to die. In this family everybody was always anxious about the health of the other family members. It could be regarded as a family with an anxiety neurosis. I referred them to our family therapists.

The therapists talked with the family, but they did this in a different way than I expected. They did not go into the history. For instance I knew there had been problems since the family had had to leave their own farm. There was no question of psychological or psychiatric assessments. They only focused on how these people interacted with one another and they gave them instructions in this respect. Sometimes even paradoxical orders. The symptoms and complaints of Mrs. Poppy were for instance encouraged, but she was instructed to express these only on certain days of the week while on other days she was not allowed to talk about them. (In this way they hoped to teach her to get more grip on her symptoms.) I had often felt that beneath the surface sweetness of Mrs. Poppy a hard kernel was concealed and that she could be very dominating in her family and in a certain way also in her relationship with me. But I had not seen what the family therapists spotted immediately i.e. that Mrs. Poppy made everybody powerless and delicately checkmated her helpers by keeping or worsening her complaints. The family therapists thwarted her in turn by stating in the very first interview that they realized that she was in such a bad state that they did not think they would be able to help her. The only thing they could try to do was help Mrs. Poppy and her family to live with her symptoms.

As could be foreseen Mrs. Poppy did not like this pronouncement. She revolted and a heavy struggle for power started between her and the therapists. In her distress she called more and more often upon me, the priest, the neighbours and relatives. The telephone in my house rang day and night and even my patient secretary almost lost her temper. Mrs. Poppy tried to escape by demanding to be referred to a psychiatrist but after consultation with the family therapists I refused to do this. She frightened her family and neighbours more and more and began to threaten with suicide. The family therapists took this very seriously and talked at length with her over the way she was going to do this, how and where, what kind of dress she would be wearing and so on. They asked her about the burial ceremony she wanted and what she thought about the impact on her family. Mrs. Poppy went through hell but to my astonishment and great relief shortly afterwards came out of it as though re-born. Since then she and her family have calmed down and steadied on to a lasting healthier course. The last move of the family therapists was to express in their final session with the family that they surely expected relapses.

Mrs. Vetchling I knew from her youth. As a girl she had a difficult time when she discovered that she had been born before her mother married a widower with several children and that her own father was unknown. She was married now herself and had a nice boy of three. Her husband was of an agreable character and had a good job. They had a new house and seemed to prosper when Mrs. Vetchling started to indulge in alcoholic dissipations. She ruined the furniture then and I was called several times and found a complete chaos in the house. After these excesses she always repented and made apologies but nevertheless this behaviour was repeated time and again. Her liver function tests deteriorated. Her husband did his best to keep her from drinking, he removed all bottles and took care that she did not have the money to buy new ones. He was worried about the impact of his wife's behaviour on their son and for this reason he was not willing to think about a second baby.

The family therapist to whom I referred Mrs. Vetchling chose a strategy I had not expected. He was struck by the way Mr. Vetchling "handed in" his wife and noticed that he adressed her as a child while she called him daddy (both of them were 32 years old). He ordered Mr. Vetchling to stop all efforts to keep his wife from drinking and he even encouraged her to drink. It transpired that when she had taken alcohol she started to abuse her husband, apologizing for this afterwards and not being able to repeat what she had said in her drunkenness. The family therapist tempted her abuses and succeeded in getting problems between the spouses out in the open. He encouraged her agressiveness and in this way made it possible to discuss their mutual relationship. Serious problems in communication between husband and wife appeared to exist, covered by the symptoms of her alcoholic behaviour. Mrs. Vetchling stopped drinking and some time ago I helped her to deliver her second baby. All went very smoothly and harmoniously. I was struck by the exclamation of "daddy" at the heigth of her labour, but I noticed that he answered her with "mammy". Of course we will have to wait and see how things will be in the future, but at this moment the relationship between the couple seems to have bettered considerably.

By these sketchy case histories I hope to have illustrated that family therapy proved to be a kind of adventure for us general practitioners. I often held my breath and was impressed by the risks that were taken. The family therapists challenged and rated our patients higher then we were used to doing as their general practitioners.

What we learned
I will now try to summarize what we learned in our cooperation with family therapists.
— Family therapy is a therapy of relationships, especially of those between members of a small group of people living together. It is not important whether this is a family in the traditional sense or not. Sometimes the sessions take place with a couple of partners, sometimes with a complete family and sometimes with a whole network of relations. Variations and improvisations are possible. In the beginning we had to motivate and refer complete families but this raised opposition and gave us problems. Later on we discovered that things went better when we referred the individuals, who came for help to the general practitioner, to the family therapist for an acquaintance, leaving it up to him to draw in other persons and to motivate them for therapy. The family therapist will always strive to involve those relevant in his therapy. It also proved to be possible to draw the general practitioner, the social worker, the minister and other professional helpers into the sessions. There is much room for improvisation, dependent on individual circumstances and possibilities. Our therapists sometimes visited the families in their own homes, but to make supervision possible a large part of the sessions had to take place behind a one way vision screen. This brought about far less objection from our patients than we had anticipated.

— We learned that to motivate our patients for this kind of therapy, it was better to start from the worries *about* symptoms and the *consequences* of disturbances having implications for the other family members, then to start from a search of *causes* of these disturbances in the family. This last line creates resistance and leads to fruitless theoretical discussions. The kind of disturbances treated can range from purely organic disease to psychological problems. The question of the cause of the disturbance can better be left open.

— The family therapists started and worked with "here and now" phenomena. They worked with these in a way that could be watched and commented upon by everybody concerned. Endless and ineffective talk about important absentees (usual in conventional individual psychotherapy) is out of the question. Nobody is excluded, but neither is anyone forced to participate if he does not wish to do so.

— Our family therapists worked with very limited numbers of sessions after which they referred the patients back to the g.p. with instructions on how to proceed. So there appeared to be no danger of new fixations and addictions, so well known in traditional psychotherapy. They strove for a short treatment, never more than a few months, but emphasized the possibility of a renewed contact if that proved necessary. In this way people were not fixated in their patient role but were given back their own responsibility as soon as possible.

— The best moments to refer to family therapy proved to be times of crises. At these moments our patients were motivated to accept help and the probability of being able to bring about changes proved to be greatest. We learned that family therapists often intentionally provoked crises, making cooperation between therapist and family doctor indispensable to prevent conflicting lines of conduct in the treatment of these families. Often it will be necessary to agree in dividing the different roles in the strategy of approach between family therapist and family doctor. Our family therapists accepted the consequence and were on call for crises intervention also during nights and weekends.

— The cooperation with the family therapists has taught us to look more intensively at families. What is the structure of this family, in what phase of development, with which specific problems? How is the communication between the family members? Do they speak straight-forwardly to one another and in the first person or obliquely via a third party and more *about* themselves and others? What about the messages they are sending and receiving, are these clear and without possibilities of misconception or are these ambiguous and internally conflicting? Above all it is important to ask oneself whether symptoms and illnesses are used as hidden messages. How far do the members let one another free, which are their rules and mutual myths? Is change and growth, differentiation and autonomy of the individual members allowed? The family therapists taught us to be more

138

on the alert to these things, and to make a better use of our home visits to do observations.

— Takig all things into consideration, our experiences with family therapy have been very favourable. The way of thinking and acting of family therapists and family doctors are in certain respects much alike. We are glad to have found one another and we have learned that by cooperation in a short time changes for the better can sometimes be brought about, even in families which we regarded as hopeless and where other helping professionals had failed.

Evaluation

Up till now I have only been speaking about subjective impressions and experiences. But we also made an endeavour to measure successes and failures. Medical students chose at random five families referred to the family therapists from each of the six practices that referred most families. They also selected from each practice five matched-controlled families, resembling the referred families as closely as possible in age of the parents, date of marriage, social level, religion, number and age of the children. The records of these families were scrutinized, all contacts with the family doctor, referrals to specialists, number and kind of prescriptions were counted during one year before and after the moment of referral to the family therapists. Two families are not included because they moved to another place. Figures 33 and 34 give the results of the addition of the numbers of contacts with the general practitioner and of the prescriptions per month. In both figures there is a marked and significant (signtest p $<0,01$) difference between the problem and control families during the year before referral. In the year following family therapy both the lines of the control families remain on the same level, but these of the problem families tend to go down. The difference between before and after referral reaches no statistical significance for the contacts with the g.p., but it does so (p $<0,02$) for the number of prescriptions. In the number of referrals to specialists there were no significant differences between before and after referral for family therapy, but these numbers were small.

To deepen my insight I studied the records of the first 26 families referred for family therapy in my own practice. I included in this the six families which broke off the contact with the therapist after one or a few sessions. Table XVI,1 gives the numbers of these 26 families.

Applying the Wilcoxon matched-pairs signed-ranks test, we learn that the differences between the period of 12 months before and 3 months after referral (= during treatment) are not significant, but those between 12 months before and after the completion of family therapy are significant (*** $\alpha = 0,01$; ** $\alpha = 0,005$; * $0,05<\alpha<0,10$) for total number of contacts, number of diagnoses and number of nervous disorders. This makes it very

139

Table 16.1 medical data of 26 families (comprising 116 individuals) in my practice referred for family therapy

time span in respect to date of referral	number of contacts with g.p.	number of diagnoses		number of prescriptions		referrals to spec.	admission into hospital
		totals	nerv. dis orders	totals	psycho- active drugs		
12 months before	619	307	53	609	184	12	1
1th-3rd month after (multiplied by 4)	604	292	32	672	224	20	0
4th-15th month after	478***	253**	28*	539	160	23	3

probable that the family therapy helped to make these families at least more self-reliant.

Further analysis showed that the number of contacts with the g.p. diminished significantly not only for the identified patient but also for the rest of the family members ($\alpha = 0,01$). The same was true ($\alpha = 0,05$) for the total number of prescriptions of psychoactive drugs ($0,05 < \alpha < 0,10$). These last findings make it plausible that something happened in the therapy not only with the patients who gave rise to these referrals but also with their families.

I realize that these figures are small, but the data collected are "harder" than usual in this kind of research. All of these point in the same direction: a diminution in the seeking of medical help. I think this to be a hopeful sign.

Our family therapists also tried to evaluate what they were doing. They sent evaluation forms to general practitioners and families 9 months after the termination of their therapy. Of the first 102 families asked to do so, 71% returned the filled in formula, while all g.p.'s answered. There proved to be no difference between the responding and non-responding families in social level or kind of problems reported at referral. Neither were there differences in the way of ending therapy (finished or broken off) or in succes rate as reported by the general practitioner. The g.p.'s thought the problems to have bettered in 56% of the families, while the medical demands had lessened in 45%, had remained stable in 50% and had increased in 5%. The numbers of prescriptions had decreased in 42%, remained the same in 57% and increased in 1%.

The families themselves said that in more than half of them the problems had disappeared or bettered, while they had remained the same in a quarter. Of those in which problems still existed almost three quarters stated that they had learned to live with them and were not troubled any more.

140

Fig. 33. Number of contacts with general practitioner before and after referral for family therapy.

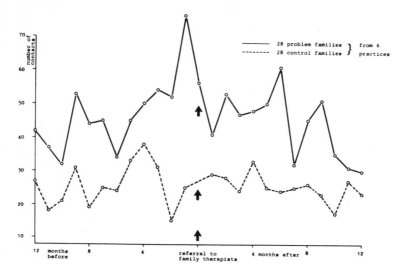

Fig. 34. Number of prescriptions before and after referral for family therapy.

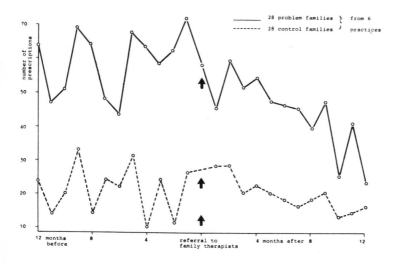

What do these findings mean?

If we realize that the average number of sessions with these families was only four, comprising a span of about two months, it can be said that these results confirmed our hope of family therapy as a short and rather simple form of therapy, suitable for application in primary health care. Since I started the cooperation with family therapists I have never found it necessary to refer patients to psychiatrists or agencies of mental health care.

The effects of family therapy have been satisfactory for most of the patients and the general practitioners. Of course we will have to keep in mind that spontaneous recovery is often taking place in psychotherapy, as stressed for instance by Truax and Carkhuff (1967). Nevertheless I think that our pilot studies confirm the view that it can be profitable to regard the family as a unit of operation in our efforts to combat illness, unhealthiness and unhappiness. The results seem to indicate that this can lead at least to a furthering of the independence from health professionals of the small group in which humans live together and grow up.

In the future we will continue to cooperate with family therapists. The question arises as to whether family therapy can be practised by the family doctor himself. In the past I have been inclined to answer this question in a negative sense, thinking this could bring him into serious role conflicts. At the moment I am not so certain about this. Every family doctor can learn a good deal from family therapy. Some of these attainments he will be able to apply in his daily practice. Straight forward, methodical family therapy, however, will always ask for abilities that can only be acquired by serious study and training under supervision of experts in this field. I do not see why a family doctor should not be able to achieve this.

References:

Comley, A. (1973), Canadian Family Physician, 19, 78-81.
Tomm, K. (1973), Canadian Family Physician, 19, 51-60.
Truax, C. and R. Carkhuff, Toward effective counseling and psychotherapy, training and practice, Aldine Publishing Company, Chicago 1967.

XVII. Family Medicine

Introduction

In most countries the general practitioner has always been acting as a doctor to the family. Names like "family doctor", "médecin de famille", "Familienarzt" indicate this. In Western Europe this still is so, as the family members usually have the same general practitioner. In the United States of America, Canada, in Eastern Europe and also in Southern Europe fragmentation of medical care of the family has been brought about by the independent growth of pediatrics, gynecology and internal medicine, also by the development of different systems of organization of health care.

It seems a remarkable fact that the United States, where the allround general practitioner was threatened most seriously with extinction, became the first country to recognize the general practitioner as a specialist in his own right, on the same level as other specialists. Calling this specialty "family medicine" however has caused a serious confusion of nomenclature, clearly brought out by Ransom and Vandervoort in their article, "The Development of Family Medicine" (1973). They rightly point out that the terms "family practice" and "family medicine" mean different things that need to be clearly distinguished. "Family practice" is a recognized medical speciality in the U.S., representing a model of primary health care closely resembling the ideals of general practice in Western Europe. Ransom and Vandervoort define this as follows: "It is a discipline of synthesis, integrating a wide range of medical and personal skills into the practice of a single physician. In theory family practice means comprehensive, continuing care provided to all age groups by a personal physician".

Most North American medical schools have developed departments giving a training in this specialty. It is however evident that this development originated with the desire to face the crisis in primary health care in the U.S., trying to counteract the overspecialized and predominantly episodic character of health care. The term "family medicine" was used (by medical schools, the authorities and the medical profession) to give new life and attraction to a dying out profession, but one which the public badly needed. In reality the education in this "specialty" has little to do with the family or with family medicine as a scientific discipline in its own right.

143

One could add that the confusion of names has been aggravated still more by the arrival of "family therapy", practised mostly by psychiatrists, social scientists and social workers.

What is meant by the expression "Family Medicine"?

In elucidating what is meant by "family practice" and "family medicine" we can distinguish between family medicine as a function, — the being of a family practitioner — and family medicine as a scientific discipline, with its own study objectives and its own methods.

Family medicine as a function is being practised in large parts of the Western world by general practitioners in that they are mostly functioning as doctors of families. Perhaps one could even argue that this should be the specific function of general practitioners as no other doctor is doing this in the same way. It enables the g.p. to make observations of family life denied to other medical practitioners, especially as only he makes home visits. He will then often see the whole family together at home, i.e. at mealtimes or at night. These visits often take place at crucial times — lying-in periods, times of stress caused by serious disease or accidents, or during domestic rows. He knows from experience that families differ markedly, not only in composition and structure, but also in phase of development, internal climate and in interaction both within the family and with the social surroundings — specifically in their inclination to call in his help. An experienced general practitioner knows a great deal about families in an unscientific context and he reckons with this in his diagnosis, his therapy and his management. This knowledge differs from scientific knowledge which "is concerned with observation and classification of facts especially with the establishment of verifiable general laws, chiefly by induction and hypotheses" (Webster's Collegiate Dictionary, 5th edition).

Family medicine as a scientific discipline is only beginning to emerge. At what point may an independent branch of science be said to be established? The most obvious criteria are the presence of its own objectives of knowledge and the application of its own methods. In medicine the criteria for acknowledgment as a discipline in its own right are hard to define. In its foundation and education medicine has always leaned heavily on physics and chemistry and other "auxiliary" sciences; and the methods used in investigation and therapy are the same in different branches of medicine. In his plea for recognition of general practice as an academic discipline I.M. Richardson (U.K., 1975) supported by a Leading Article (1975, in the Lancet) puts forward four criteria. First, the kind of morbidity treated must be definable and of sufficient quantity. Secondly, skills have to be taught in defining and solving problems which differ from those of other disciplines. Thirdly, there has to be a recognizable philosophy, a point of view; and fourthly the discipline must create and support active research. It is remarkable that in this context the author does not even mention family

144

medicine, although he often speaks about the family doctor.

I am strongly in favour of regarding family medicine as an emerging academic discipline. This can be defined as Ransom and Vandervoort do: "Family medicine is an emerging discipline concerned with the relationship of life in small groups to health, illness and care. Its focus is on the ecology of relations among individuals in families and between families and their surrounding environment". They stress that "family medicine embodies a fundamental shift in point of view toward health and illness and strategies of intervention". In their opinion the most important factor in family medicine is the way of looking at health and disease. This has already been stated very clearly by the American father of family medicine H.B. Richardson, who in his book "Patients have families" wrote as long ago as 1945: "The idea of disease as an entity which is limited to one person, and can be transmitted or spread from one individual to another, fades into the background, and disease becomes an integral part of the continuous process of living. The family is the unit of illness, because it is the unit of living".

It could be argued that family medicine promotes a way of thinking about health and illness with revolutionary consequences. H.B. Richardson was an American physician, whose points of view have been developed further mostly by psychiatrists and social scientists. This led to the emergence of family therapy. But Richardson and his co-workers took a broader view. They gave impetus to the development of family medicine in a wide sense, so that it encompassed both psychological problems and somatic disorders. Family medicine in this broad sense has not yet been developed as a discipline in its own right, but important foundations have been laid by social scientists, family doctors, pediatricians and psychiatrists.

Basic Conceptions of Family Medicine

In this last chapter of my book I will try to consider those conceptions that seem to me to be of basic importance for the development of family medicine as a discipline.

What is a family?

One of the major causes of misunderstanding and possibly resistance against the development of a broad family medicine is the misconception that this term implies as its goal the promotion, defence and maintenance of the traditional form of the nuclear family as we know it in the West. In fact the contrary could be argued; for the most vehement critics of this kind of family have come from family therapists and social scientists interested in family life.

The meaning of the word "family" has to be taken much more broadly than comprising a married couple with children. It is used for any small group in which people live together, eat and sleep together, whatever

145

composition, form or name the group may have. The only important thing in the definition of "family" is that this small group has its own common past and future, although these may be of limited duration. Probably more than 90% of all people in the Western world live in such small family groups. Most have the character of husband and wife with their children, but this is not an essential feature. Small groups of only men or women, concubinates and communes, with or without children, can be regarded as families if the composition is not purely accidental and if the arrangement is not merely a temporary expedient.

Even the boundaries of "family" do not always coincide with living together. Often key figures living elsewhere have such a strong influence on the small group that they have to be regarded as being in fact part of the family system.

The family as a unit

The essence of family medicine (and of family therapy) is to regard not the human individual but the family as the unit of action. That is the level of application. The family is regarded as more than the sum of its individual members; just as an organism is more than a collection of organs, and an organ more than an agglomeration of cells. The individual family members are involved with one another in several ways: they communicate, they influence one another, and are interdependent. Every change in one causes changes in each of the others, and in the family as a whole. This conception has far-reaching consequences for the physician who has learned in his training — at best — to think of individuals who have diseases. It seems to be very difficult for him to change this. Nevertheless the ability to identify the family as a unit or system is "sine qua non" in the development of family medicine. I have tried to do this in presenting the case histories in this book, but it is evident that I have only partly succeeded.

Certain parallels can be shown with biology: a family has structures like an organism, it also shows life processes such as growth, differentiation and involution; it has its own life cycle and its own functions.

Homoiostasis and *steady state* are familiar concepts in physiology and medicine. Like a living organism, the family strives to maintain its internal equilibrium and to maintain a balanced relationship with the environment. This does not mean stagnation, as exchanges of energy to and fro are continually taking place. At the same time the system tries to preserve its status. It is important to recognize this in family medicine. Changes provoke counteraction. The getting well of one family member may result in illness of another. Growth and development of the individual family members are modified by the family system. When the development of the family is "sound", a gradual differentiation and development of the personality — individuation — of its members take place, yet the system as a whole still tends to preserve its equilibrium.

In medicine the term "homoiostasis" has a favourable meaning, but in family therapy it is inappropriate. Family therapists strongly believe in the value of flexibility. It is true that the family system can inhibit the individual development of its members, but on the other hand a too rapid disparity among one or more members can lead to disorders in the family or even in the system itself.

Symbiosis also does not have a pejorative meaning in biology. It is used to characterize a living together of two dissimilar organisms which need but do not harm one another. However, in family dynamics symbiotic means: preventing individuation. "Enmeshment" and "undifferentiated ego mass" mean much the same thing. In these families everybody is constantly concerned with everybody else. The "we"-feeling of the family members in relation to the outer world is too strong, and there are no divisions between the members of the family. I described an example of this kind of family in chapter II and XVI. Every family doctor will know such families from experience. Their members tend to call the doctor more for one of the others than for themselves. They are over-anxious for one another: the husband calls the doctor for his wife, the wife for her husband, the children for their parents and vice versa. In these families the children experience great difficulties in freeing themselves from the system as they grow up.

The expression *family crisis* also varies in meaning. It is used to denote all situations in which the family has to adapt to changes — such as the birth of a child, going off to school and later leaving school, the wife taking a job, moving into another house, retirement etc. In family crises the probability of illness and disorders of its members is increased.

Family rules. In every kind of society rules are indispensable. We know that in every small group (even in the transitory roleplaying of strangers) rules soon emerge and develop spontaneously. A family doctor should be prepared for this phenomenon when trying to help families, otherwise he may encounter unexpected resistance. Mores and taboos are very important in family life. Changing of these can give rise to family crises.

Health and disease have a somewhat different meaning in family medicine than that usually understood by physicians treating individuals. As Richardson has already stated in his book, symptoms and signs of illness are an inherent part of human life. Last ("The Iceberg of Disease" 1963) and many others have shown that most "healthy" people usually have several complaints, either bodily or mental. The study of the 200 families mentioned in chapter XV brought this to light. These symptoms and complaints are extremely important in daily life and in human interactions. In the family context one has to focus not merely on individual symptoms or diseases, but on the influence of these on the other members and on the family as a whole. The interactions within the family in the field of health and disease are of prime interest in family medicine. An individual has need of others not only to live healthily, but also to be able to be ill. Most illnesses are dealt with by the family itself; only for a minority (10-20%) is professional medical help called in. In family medicine it is extremely important to learn how families handle symptoms and disease, and whether this is functional or dysfunctional to family life. Special note should be taken of the way the family members behave with one another.

When a personal physician is confronted with symptoms of disease he is strongly inclined to do two things almost immediately: try to find a (personal) cause and to apply specific treatment. A family physician's approach is fundamentally different: he will assess the effects of the symptoms of illness, not only on the individual patient, but also on the other members and the family as a whole. He will consider what they mean, what their function is and how they are manipulated in the family. Furthermore he will not confine his attention to causes within the individual but will also look for causes arising in the family as a whole. Perhaps the most important difference is that he is less inclined to interfere — in case he might risk suppressing meaningful symptoms, hampering family processes and making the family dependent on him. Rather he will encourage the family to find its own solutions. Sometimes he will even accentuate the symptoms of one member, hoping to elicit counter-reactions ("paradoxical therapy").

Circular causation

The differences in thinking go still further. In family medicine multicausal thinking is more pronounced. The realization is always present that a phenomenon may have several causes and a single cause may have several effects. This fits in well with modern trends in medical thinking. We know that the origins of many diseases are complex and that the human organism is capable of giving only a limited number of responses to given stimuli. The difference in thinking about causation goes however deeper. In his training the physician is taught to think about causation mainly in linear terms, i.e. A causes B, B causes C, etc.:

$$A \rightarrow B \rightarrow C.$$

A knowledge of family dynamics enables one to see that there is always a reciprocal action between A, B and C:

$$A \leftrightarrow B \leftrightarrow C$$

Almost always the behaviour of A is partly determined by the wishes or provocations of B.

Often in a family the causation is of a circular kind i.e.: A causes B, B causes C, but C causes A in its turn:

$$A \leftrightarrow B$$
$$\nwarrow_C \nearrow$$

And it may be very difficult and also irrelevant in family dynamics to tell

148

what is the primary cause. In larger families when subgroup formation is taking place, the interactions are still more complicated.

The Identified Patient

A physician, called in by a patient, is usually inclined to react without first asking himself how far this "patient" is being pushed forward by a (family) system. In fact he himself may unwittingly become an extension of the family in this way and often indeed is an integral part of family mechanisms. I have often fallen into this trap, as I have described in some of the case histories. Once his eyes are opened the doctor will come to realize that this sequence of events is happening more often than he thought, and in this way he can actually promote and stabilize family pathology. The most obvious example is the family scapegoat; but this may easily pass unrecognized because the scapegoat himself is playing an active part in maintaining the balance within the family, merely by assuming the role of scapegoat (see circular causation). This interplay within the family is not confined to psychiatric and behavioural disorders, but occurs also in the course of physical disease.

Comprehensive Medicine

Family therapy is directed mainly to psycho-social disorders. In his book "The Efficiency of Medical Care" Prof. Querido (1955) has established beyond doubt that all kinds of interaction exist between the somatic, psychological and social fields. A disorder in one of the fields can manifest itself in another and be treated in still another field. Querido's book was the result of an investigation of individuals. What he proved to be true in human individuals is even more true in families. The interactions within and between the physical field (genetics, housing, food, infections etc.), the psychological field (awareness of one's self and others) and social field (habits, norms and rules) are even more obvious in a family.

Really broad-based family medicine must be concerned not only with the psycho-social aspect but with the total health care of the family. In mental health care, family therapy is rapidly gaining ground. In physical health care, almost all therapy is of an individual nature; but in this field also a family approach should be cultivated, not only in the context of treatment, but also — and more especially — in the contexts of support and prevention. The independence, emancipation and responsibility of the small human group will have to be safeguarded and encouraged. In doing so a considerable part of what is being treated now in hospitals and institutions could be dealt with at home. The "medicalization of society" (Illich 1975), which is rapidly taking place, could be countered in this way. Our conventional health care is making people progressively more dependent upon professional help. Perhaps the greatest challenge for family medicine is to recognize and make use of the active participation of the small group. This applies to physical disease and disability as well. This development has hardly started. Strategies will have to be designed and tested. Perhaps the achievements of family therapy can show the way.

The Principle of Risk Assessment
In every branch of medicine it is very important to be able to assess risks and to foresee what is likely to happen. In fact a prognosis is more important than a diagnosis, and certainly this is a better justification of therapy. In family medicine the art and science of assessing risks will have to be further developed. It seems useful to assess the balance between the ability of families to carry burdens of life on the one hand, and the burdens to be carried on the other. For a family doctor it is not so difficult to assess the burdens of life, but the assessment of the ability to carry them calls for an altogether new insight. In chapter XV I indicated the direction in which we at our Institute are investigating. Much more research will have to be done before we are on firm ground and before we can translate our findings into something useful for general practitioners.

In this chapter I have tried to describe some concepts that seem to be important in the formation and development of family medicine. I have been far from complete and I realize that the conclusions I have reached may to others seem wrong or irrelevant. In my opinion this does not matter much as long as the reader is stimulated to think and to read further for himself about the challenging subject of family medicine as an emergent discipline.

Some practical suggestions
I will end this last chapter with some practical suggestions which might perhaps help general practitioners to reach the family level in their thinking. We have learned that in aiming at medicine of the whole person and at a complete diagnosis it is imperative to ask oneself when consulted by a patient: why does this particular individual ask my help at this particular moment for this particular symptom or illness? In a similar way, we can ask ourselves the following questions before proceeding further.
1. — *What do I know of the family origins?* In my case histories I have given many examples of the importance of heridity in physical disease and of the far-reaching consequences of the social conditions in which children are brought up.
2 — *What do I know of the family he or she is living in?* — its composition and *structure*. Is it a complete or incomplete family? Are there subgroups discernable? The solidarity between the members of the family unit is important especially between those of the same generation and it is usually harmful when coalitions are formed between children and one of the parents, opposing other members.

150

— In what *phase of development* is this family in its life cycle? A family changes in composition and character in the course of its existence. Usually four or five phases are discerned: the *first* is of a young couple without children; the *second* of the family with young children; the *third*, families with children going to school and leaving home; the *fourth*, the "empty nest" family and the *last* phase is retirement and old age. Each of these phases brings different and specific problems with them and especially transitions of one phase into the next demand adaptions and changes. Often disturbances arise because old solutions are tried for new situations and problems.

— *What about its internal and external relationships and communications?* The emotional bonds and the interactions between the members and with the surrounding community are of special importance. What kind of rules do they have? What is the internal climate?

3 — *What do I know of the medical and social history of this family?* Which diseases and problems have they presented in the past? What about their illness behaviour and their coping capabilities? A general practitioner usually will know a good deal about this.

4 — *What does this particular individual symptom of illness with which I am confronted mean in this particular family?* Does it express something or point to specific causes? What are the consequences for this family? What do they think and what did they do themselves about it? Will they be able to cope?

5 — *Which will be the impact of my modes of action regarding this problem on this particular family?* By his frequent contacts with the same families in the course of time the general practitioner exerts an influence on the health and life of these families that must not be underestimated.

Perhaps these five questions can be of some help to general practitioners in their daily work as an aid in focusing on the level of the family unit.

References:
Illich, I. (1975), Medical Nemesis, Calder-Boyars Ltd., London.
Last, J.M. (1963), The iceberg, completing the clinical picture in general practice, The Lancet, vol. 2, 28.
Leading article (1975), Academic general practice. Br. Med. J. 4: 724.
Querido, A. (1963), The efficiency of medical care. H.S. Stenfert Kroese n.v., Leiden.
Ransom, D.A. and H.E. Vandervoort (1973), The development of family medicine-problematic trends, JAMA 225: 1098.
Richardson, H.B. (1945), Patients have families; 3rd pr. New York, Commonwealth Fund, p. 76.
Richardson, I.M. (1975), The value of a university department of general practice. Br. Med. J. 4: 740.

Conclusion

This book started with case-studies of the medical life history of families which illustrated the importance of family life in maintaining healthy members. Out of this arose the thesis that a general practitioner should regard the family as an important unit in his daily work. This thesis was supported subsequently by analysing statistical evidence gathered in family surveys.

Readers of this book might misconstrue its contents. Perhaps some will think that the case-histories represent a selection of the most ill in my practice, but they would be wrong. Of course it is true that they were selected, but I could have given dozens of other examples and some even more seriously ill. Perfectly healthy families do not exist. In the life of every family episodes of illness play a role and no family leads a continuously harmonious existence. As a matter of fact I believe I could write a story about nearly every one of the thousand families in my practice. Numerous investigations all over the world have proved that "healthy" people generally have several symptoms and signs of disease. In 1975 our family therapists interviewed a number of inconspicuous families who regarded themselves as healthy and happy. They had been invited as volunteers to explore "normal families". It appeared that in most of them several — sometimes serious — problems were discovered.

A reader's further misunderstanding could be to suppose that my practice consists of very unhealthy and unhappy families. Really they are a prosperous and reasonably happy population. The mortality figures in my practice for many years have been about 10% below those of the country as a whole. The definition of health by the World Health Organization as a state of complete physical, mental and social well-being is a misleading and unrealistic fiction. Illness, death, mishaps and unhappiness are with us at all times and a family doctor witnesses this, although he sees only part of it. Several investigations in the Netherlands and in the United Kingdom have shown that on the average a general practitioner is called upon at least once in every year by about 80%, and in four years by almost 100% of all "normal" families in his practice. The numbers of consultations per individual per year in my practice are about half of the average for the country.

152

A third misunderstanding, this time regarding the family surveys in this book, would be to assume that the results of these can be extrapolated to other populations and other family doctors, but they can only hold true for my practice and my country. Although the findings are in agreement with those of similar studies in different countries (see Cohen, Yofe and Davies 1960, Hare and Shaw 1965, Buck and Laughton 1959, Marinker 1969, Picken and Ireland 1969, Polliack 1971), much more research will have to be done in this difficult but fascinating field. The significance of the family in the passing on, expanding and preserving of human life, setting standards essential in physical, psychological and social spheres seems to me to be of such great importance — and will probably continue to be so in the near future — that it merits more investigation, preferable multi-disciplinary. I hope that this will open up new ways of preventing some of the things I have been describing in this book, such as the transmission of unnecessary unhappinesss and unhealthiness from generation to generation.

In this book I have tried to set down facts and views I have learned from my practice families while serving them as their doctor, facts and views which might be useful to present and future family doctors and other professionals who deal with families. The answer as to whether I have successfully done so lies with my readers. I hope they will agree with my ultimate aim in writing this book; to further the care for the well-being of family life everywhere.

References:
Buck, C.W. AND K.B. Laughton (1959), Family patterns of illness. The effect of psychoneurosis in the parent upon illness in the child, Acta Psych. Neurolog. Scandin. 34, 165.
Cohen, J., J. Yofe and A.M. Davies (1960), Family morbidity; a suggested method of measurement, Brit. J. prev. soc. Med. 14, p. 39-43.
Hare, E.H. and G.K. Shaw (1965), A study in family health; health in relation to family size. Brit. J. psych., 111, 461 and 467.
Marinker, M.L. (1969), The general practitioner as family doctor. J. Roy. Coll. Gen. Practit. 17, p. 227-236.
Picken, P. and G. Ireland (1969), Family-patterns of medical care utilization. Possible influences of family-size, role and social class of illness-behaviour. J. chron. diseases, 22, 181.
Polliack, M.R. (1971), The relationship between Cornell Medical Index scores and attendance roles. J. Roy. Coll. Gen. Practit. 21, p. 453-459.

Appendix I

Table XI,1. Some data of the 100 younger families

number of families	:	100
observation period	:	from date of marriage to 1-1-65
date of marriage	:	1945-1948

mean couple's age at marriage

-24	:	7
25-30	:	41
31-36	:	38
37-40	:	9
41-50	:	5

number of live-born children: 378, average 3.8
(0 = 12, 1 = 5, 2 = 18, 3 = 15, 4 = 10, 5 = 15, 6 = 13, 7 = 2, 8 = 7, 9 = 2, 11 = 1)
average number of children in families with children: 4.3 observed span of childbearing (the years from birth of first to last child)

1-5 years	:	26
6-10 years	:	38
11-15 years	:	22
16-20 years	:	3

number of family members who died during observation period: 11 (fathers 2, mothers 0, children 9)
number of patient-years observed: 8412

Table XI,2. correlation coefficients between numbers of diagnoses between fathers, mothers and children in 100 younger families.

fathers and mothers	:	r = 0.217	*	(p <0.05)
fathers and children	:	r = 0.298	**	(p <0.01)
mothers and children	:	r = 0.45	**	(p <0.01)

Table XI,3. Kendall's similarity-coefficients W applying the Friedman's method to the numbers of diagnoses and consultations of 4 consecutive periods of 4 years of 100 younger families.

	n	number of diagnoses per year	number of consultations per year
mothers	100	0.632***	0.529***
fathers	100	0.635***	0.531***
children	86	0.637***	0.527***
families	100	0.691***	0.559***

*** = p <0.001

Table XI.4. Spearman correlation-coëfficients between numbers of diagnoses and consultations per year in consecutive periods of 4 years in 100 younger families

mothers (no = 100)	period 1	2	3	4
Cons./year → diagn./year				
2- 5 year of marriage = 1		0.569***	0.338**	0.351**
6- 9 year of marriage = 2	0.452***		0.568***	0.535***
10-13 year of marriage = 3	0.236**	0.377***		0.702***
14-17 year of marriage = 4	0.290**	0.275**	0.602***	diagn./year
			cons./year	

fathers (no = 100)	period 1	2	3	4
cons./year → diagn./year				
2- 5 year of marriage = 1		0.574***	0.438***	0.370***
6- 9 year of marriage = 2	0.557***		0.585***	0.449***
10-13 year of marriage = 3	0.302**	0.376***		0.662***
14-17 year of marriage = 4	0.316**	0.268**	0.430***	

children (no of families = 86)	period 1	2	3	4
cons./year → diagn./year				
2- 5 year of marriage = 1		0.618***	0.379**	0.317**
6- 9 year of marriage = 2	0.566***		0.535***	0.613***
10-13 year of marriage = 3	0.208*	0.309**		0. 635***
14-17 year of marriage = 4	0.166	0.420***	0.544***	

families (no = 100)	period 1	2	3	4
cons./year → diagn./year				
2- 5 year of marriage = 1		0.672***	0.468***	0.450***
6- 9 year of marriage = 2	0.579***		0.614***	0.574***
10-13 year of marriage = 3	0.261*	0.385***		0.749***
14-17 year of marriage = 4	0.325**	0.417***	0.505*00	

Table XI. 5.

number of children	number of families with the incidence of disorders in the children	
	below median	above median
1, 2 or 3	15	23
4 or more	29	21
totals	44	44

chi-square = 2.27   d.f. = 1   0.10 < p < 0.20

Table XI, 6.

mother	number of families with the incidence of disorders in the children	
	below median	above median
stable	22	11
unstable	22	33
totals	44	44

chi-square = 4.85   d.f. = 1   0.025 < p < 0.05

Table XI, 7.

parents	number of families with the incidence of disorders in the children	
	below median	above median
both stable	15	6
one unstable	21	16
both unstable	8	22
totals	44	44

chi-square = 11.07   d.f. = 2   0.001 < p < 0.005

Table XI, 8.

parents	number of families with the incidence of respiratory disorders of the children	
	below median	above median
both stable	16	5
one unstable	20	17
both unstable	8	22
totals	44	44

chi-square = 12.54   d.f. = 2   0.001 < p < 0.005

156

Table XI, 9.

parents	number of families with the incidence of skin disorders of the children	
	below median	above median
both stable	12	9
one unstable	21	16
both unstable	12	18
totals	45	43

chi-square = 2.29   d.f. = 2 $0.25 < p < 0.50$

Table XI, 10.

parents	number of families with the incidence of accidents of the children	
	below median	above median
both stable	14	7
one unstable	18	19
both unstable	11	19
totals	43	45

chi-square = 4.39   d.f. = 2 $0.10 < p < 0.25$

Table XI, 11

parents	number of families with the incidence of nervous disorders of the children	
	below median	above median
both stable	13	8
one unstable	26	11
both unstable	6	24
totals	45	43

chi-square = 18.27   d.f. = 2 $p < 0.0005$

Table XI, 12.

marriage - relationship	number of families with the incidence of disorders in the children	
	below median	above median
good	43	31
poor	1	13
totals	44	44

chi-square = 10.28   d.f. = 1 $0.001 < p < 0.005$

Table XII, 1.

Some data of the 100 older families

Number of families: 100
Observation period: 20 years (1-7-45 to 1-7-65)
Date of marriage: 1921-1930 (median in 1927)
wife's age at marriage: 18-46 (median at 25)
(19:7, 20-24 : 22, 25-29 : 42, 30-34 : 23, 35-39 : 2, 40-44 : 3, 45- : 1)
Husband's age at marriage: median at 28 years
Number of live-born children: 531, average = 5
(0 = 8, 1-3 = 35, 4-6 = 24, 7 or more = 33)
Observed span of childbearing (the years from birth of first to last child) average: 9 years
(1-5 years : 20, 6-10 years : 24, 11-15 years : 19, 16-20 years : 17, 21-25 years : 5, 26-30 years : 1,
1 child : 6, no children 8)
Number of family members who died during observation period : 38
(fathers 23, mothers 11, children 4)
Number of patient years observed: 10.655

Table XII, 2.	young	older
number of families	101-110	201-210
number of parents	20	20
number of children	44	49
number of patient-years	867	1030
total number of consultations	1946	2272
number of consultations per year of observation		
of all patients	2.2	2.2
of fathers	2.5	2.7
of mothers (for illness)	2.9	3.5
of mothers (for maternity care)	3.7	0.2
of all children	2.0	1.8
percentages of all consultations		
emergencies	3	2.1
referrals to specialist	4.3	4.4
admissions to hospital	2.4	1.6

Table XII, 3.	younger families	older families
number of patient-years observed	8412	10655
number of consultations (without natal care)	22470	23763
number of diagnoses	12478	10259
number of consultations per diagnosis	1.9	2.3
averages *per family per year*		
number of diagnoses	1.5	1.0
number of consultations	2.7	2.2
number of emergency consultations	0.05	0.05
number of referrals to specialist	0.07	0.07
number of admissions to hospital	0.03	0.03

Table XII, 4.
Arranging the 89 older families with children along the order of the indices for the total numbers of *diagnoses* of father, mother and children during 20 years, a very significant similarity was found with the Friedman test. In this test the Kfall's similarity-coëfficient W proved to be 0.60 (maximum of W being I, minimum 0, P < 10 $^{-4}$). Spearman's order-correlation-coefficients between the indices of the family members were:
between fathers and mothers: 0.26 (0.01 < P < 0.02)
between fathers and children: 0.49 (P < 10 $^{-3}$)
between mothersand children: 0.46 (P < 10 $^{-3}$)
All three correlation-coefficients are statistically significant, but the correlation between parents and children is much greater than that between the parents themselves.

Table XII, 5. Correlation within families of total diagnoses over 20 years in 89 older families with children by disease category.

disease category	number of instances of frequency = 0				ordercoefficient of Spearman 3)		
	M	F	Ch	W 2)	M/F	M/Ch	F/Ch
upper respiratory disord. 1)	48	48	11	0.431*	−0.019	0 186(*)	0.257*
lower respiratory disord.	21	22	6	0.528***	0.250*	0.294**	0.350**
skin and mucous membr.	16	16	0	0.564***	0.237*	0.340**	0.461***
gastro-intestinal disord.	31	37	13	0.478**	0.105	0.256*	0.281**
nervous disorders	13	40	4	0.463**	0.253*	0.165	0.170
accidents	28	30	4	0.460**	0.094	0.265*	0.210*
infective diseases 1)	86	82	43	0.346	−0.063	0.043	0.043
urogenital disorders 1)	29	74	49	0.312	−0.185(*)	0.132	−0.121
other disorders	8	7	10	0.382	0.086	0.008	0.126

(*)   statistical significance correlation-coefficient 0.05 P ≦0.10
*   statistical significance correlation-coefficient 0.01 P ≦0.05
**   statistical significance correlation-coefficient 0.001 P ≦0.01
***   statistical significance correlation-coefficient P ≦0.001
M = mother   F = father   Ch = children
1)   testing results unreliable due to too many scores being zero
2)   W = Kendall's similarity coefficient in the order of numbers of diagnoses between fathers, mothers and children
3)   in testing the correlation-coefficients their interdependance has not been taken into account

Table XII, 6. Correlation matrix of family indices for disorders of 89 older families with children (1 = disorders of lower respiratory tract, 2 = skin and mucous membranes, 3 = gastro-intestinal disorders, 4 = nervous disorders, 5 = accidents).

	1	2	3	4	5
1	1.000	0.351**	0.498**	0.379**	0.347**
2	0.351**	1.000	0.356**	0.348**	0.434**
3	0.498**	0.356**	1.000	0.291**	0.314**
4	0.379**	0.348**	0.291**	1.000	0.156
5	0.347**	0.434**	0.314**	0.156	1.000

This table shows that all correlation-coëfficients between the categories except one were significant (0.001 < P <0.01). The factor analysis gave only one factor.

Table XII, 7. Similarity of medical interactions over 20 years of 89 older families with children. With Friedmann's method of M-arrangements has been looked for significance between fathers, mothers and children of the 89 families with children. The results are presented in table XII,7. The test results are expressed in Kendall's correlation-coefficient W (max. = 1, min. = 0). The same table represents Spearman's order-correlation coefficients between numbers of activities of fathers, mothers and children.

activity	number of instances of frequence = 0			W Kendall	Spearman's order-correlation coëfficient 2)		
	M	F	Ch		M/F	M/Ch	F/Ch
normal consultations	1	0	0	0.316	−0.033	−0.070	0.024
emergency consult.	34	30	28	0.386	0.132	0.073	0.097
referrals to spec.	18	25	16	0.431*	0.132	0.111	0.245*
admissions to hosp. 1)	43	50	37	0.345	−0.082	0.205(*)	0.081

M = mother   F = father   Ch = children
(*) = doubtful significance   * = significance $0.01 < P < 0.05$
1) testing results not reliable due to too many scores being zero
2) in testing the correlation coefficients their interdependence has not been taken into account.

Tavle XII, 8. For each of the interactions (normal consultations, emergency consultations, referrals and admissions to hospital) a family index was computed, defined as: the total number of these different interactions, divided by the total number of patient-years.
The averages of these family indices were for the 100 older families:
normal consultations   2.44   (range 0.48-6.18) per patient-year
emergency consultations 1)   0.053 (range 0.00-0.17) per patient-year
referrals to specialists   0.069 (range 0.00-0.21) per patient-year
admissions to hospital   0.033 (range 0.00-0.13) per patient-year

1) for one family this figure was found to be 0.95. This was a family with an asthmatic son, requesting many emergency visits. This atypical figure has been left out. If this is not omitted the figure for emergency consultations would be: 0.062 (range 0.00-0.95). Of the 77 families for which complete social data was available, correlated with the medical data, the correlations between the four indices of interaction were computed. The family with the asthmatic boy was left out of this to avoid disturbing the correlation-coefficients. The results of the other 76 families are presented in table XII, 9.

160

Table XII, 9. Averages, standard deviations and matrix of Pearson correlation-coefficients for the family indices of:

cons. = normal consultations
ref. = referrals to specialists
adm. = admissions to hospital
st. dev. = standard deviation

76 older families	average	st. dev.	cons.	irr. cons.	ref.	adm.
cons.	2.35	1.17	1.00	0.63***	0.48***	0.19(*)
irr. cons.	0.0486	0.0370	0.63***	1.00	0.46***	0.40**
ref.	0.0616	0.0411	0.48***	0.46***	1.00	0.54***
adm.	0.0262	0.0259	0.19(*)	0.30**	0.54***	1.00

The statistical significance of the correlation-coefficients is indicated by:
(*) $0.05 < P < 0.10$
* $0.01 < P < 0.05$
** $0.001 < P < 0.01$
*** $P < 0.001$

The correlation matrix of table XII,9 has been subjected to factor analysis. In this the Jörreskog-extraction method has been used. The extraction was ended when the explained variance was more than the sum of the squares of the multiple correlation coefficients. To this criterion only one factor was of significance, explaining more than 44% of the variance. All four variables loaded more than 0.50 on this factor. On this evidence it was decided to go on with only one factor for the measures of interaction. The scores of the factor of this factor-analysis were not used, because referrals and admissions to hospital influenced this, where figures were preferred representing predominantly patient-initiated activities such as consultations and emergency consultations. To this end we chose an index representing the number of consultations — emergency consultations, divided by the number of patient-years.

For these 77 families, for which the complete social data was available, an index for diagnoses was also constructed. For this we used the sum total of the indices of diagnoses for father, mother and average child, described previously. This had the advantage (in considering the total number of diagnoses) that it was independent of the number of children. A family index, using the total number of diagnoses, would in large families be larger than in small families if all illnesses of all children were included.

Table XII,10. Spearman's correlation-coefficients, matrix of 77 older families dealing with paternal influence (p.i.), maternal influence (m.i.), psycho-social family burden (fam. burd.), material conditions (mat. cond.), year of marriage (yr. mar.), number of children (no. ch.), social class (soc. cl.), index of diagnoses (diagn. ind.) and index of consultations (cons. ind.).

no. of families 77	p.i.	m.i.	fam. burd.	mat. cond.	yr. mar.	no. ch.	soc. cl.	diagn. ind.	cons. ind.
p.i.	+ *1.00*	+ 0.05	− 0.04	− 0.14	− 0.20(*)	− 0.02	+ 0.08	− 0.13	− 0.02
m.i.	+ 0.05	+ *1.00*	+ 0.02	− 0.07	+ 0.03	− 0.16	+ 0.02	+ 0.11	+ 0.20(*)
fam. burd.	− 0.04	+ 0.02	+ *1.00*	+ 0.00	− 0.08	+ 0.21(*)	− 0.12	+ 0.22(*)	+ 0.26*
mat. cond.	− 0.14	− 0.07	+ 0.00	+ *1.00*	+ 0.12	+ 0.12	− 0.41**	+ 0.18	+ 0.03
yr. mar.	− 0.20(*)	+ 0.03	− 0.08	+ 0.12	+ *1.00*	− 0.09	− 0.08	+ 0.02	− 0.08
no. childr.	− 0.02	− 0.16	+ 0.21(*)	+ 0.12	− 0.09	+ *1.00*	+ 0.06	− 0.01	− 0.26*
soc. cl.	+ 0.08	+ 0.02	− 0.12	− 0.41**	− 0.08	+ 0.06	+ *1.00*	− 0.27*	− 0.29*
diagn. ind.	− 0.13	+ 0.11	+ 0.22(*)	+ 0.18	+ 0.02	− 0.01	− 0.27*	+ *1.00*	+ 0.72***
cons. ind.	− 0.02	+ 0.20(*)	+ 0.26*	+ 0.03	− 0.08	− 0.26*	− 0.29*	+ 0.72***	+ *1.00*

(*) $0.05 < P < 0.10$
* $0.01 < P < 0.05$
** $0.001 < P < 0.01$
*** $P < 0.001$

The left upper part of this table (first rows and columns) gives the correlations between the factors found in the factor analysis on the psycho-social data of the older families. They are low, as they should be. They would in fact have been zero, if the Pearson correlation-coefficients had been used as in the factor-analysis. The right lower part of table XII,10 (last five rows and columns) gives the correlations between the family indices for diagnoses and consultations and some social data of the families. There appears to be a very significant, but hardly surprising, correlation between the family indices for diagnoses and for consultations. It was to be expected that in families, where father, mother and children had many illnesses, the average family member would have had many consultations. The index of consultations is significantly negative correlated with social class and number of children, while the index of diagnoses shows a significant negative correlation with social class. There are no correlations with the year of marriage; the relative differences in length of marriage life between the older families does not seem to have had much influence on numbers of diagnoses and consultations.

The rest of table XII, 10 gives the relationship between the psycho-social factors and the family data. There is a very significant correlation between the factor "material conditions" and social-class — which was to be expected and which confirms that the denomination of this factor was right. A lower, but still significant, correlation is found between consultation-index and the factor "family burden". For the rest there are only weakly positive correlations between "family burden", number of live-born children and index of diagnoses and between "maternal influence" and consultation index.

Table XII, 11. Correlation matrix of Spearman's correlation-coefficients for the relationships between indices for diagnoses and consultations of fathers, mothers and children separately.
D = index of diagnoses   C = index of consultations
F = father   M = mother   Ch = children

	D.F.	D.M.	D.Ch.	C.F.	C.M.	C.Ch.
D.F.	+1.00	+0.26*	+0.48***	+0.83***	−0.02	+0.11
D.M.	+0.26*	+1.00	+0.46***	+0.32**	+0.65***	−0.07
D.Ch.	+0.48***	+0.46***	+1.00	+0.40***	+0.23*	+0.09
C.F.	+0.83***	+0.32**	+0.40***	+1.00	+0.02	+0.04
C.M.	−0.02	+0.65***	+0.23*	+0.02	+1.00	−0.07
C.Ch.	+0.11	−0.07	+0.09	+0.04	−0.07	+1.00

* $0.01 < P < 0.05$
** $0.001 < P < 0.01$
*** $P < 0.001$

N.B. The numbers of pairs for computing the correlation-coefficients are not always the same due to the occurrence of incomplete families.
These numbers were for
Fathers/Mothers   97
Fathers/Children   91
Mothers/Children   90

Table XIV, 1. Number of live-born children and social class of the families in percentages
number of children   family phase

	young	middle	old
0	—	—	5.6
1	5.7	2.5	5.6
2	5.4	20.0	16.7
3	28.6	15.0	16.7
4	11.4	7.5	5.6
5	2.9	22.5	11.1
6 and more	—	32.5	39.1
middle class	37.1	35.0	44.4
labourers	62.9	65.0	55.6
total numbers	N = 36	N = 39	N = 18

Appendix 2. Family charts

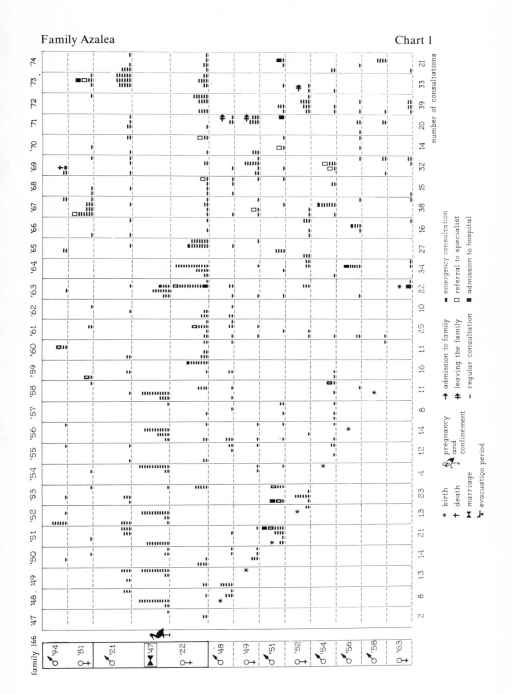

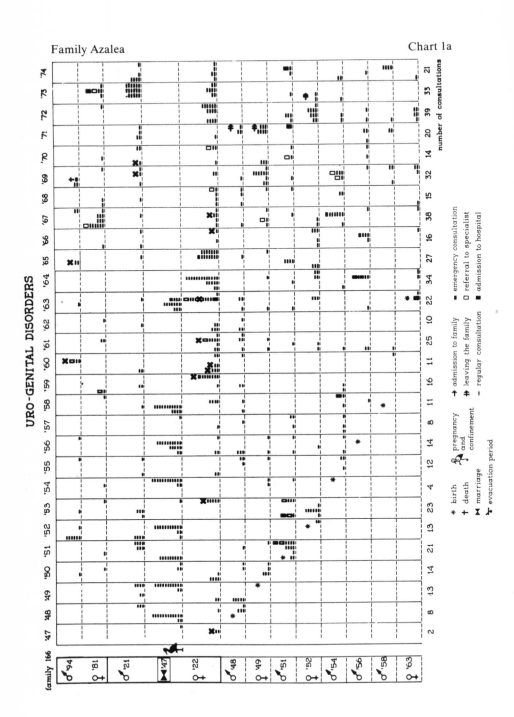

Family Azalea

URO-GENITAL DISORDERS

number of consultations

* birth
† death
✖ marriage
➤ evacuation period

🐦 pregnancy and confinement

↑ admission to family
⬆ leaving the family
– regular consultation

■ emergency consultation
□ referral to specialist
■ admission to hospital

166

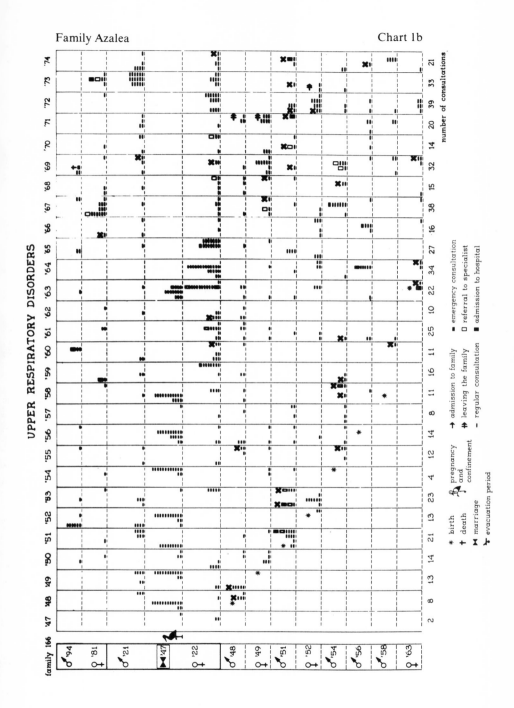

Family Azalea   Chart 1b

UPPER RESPIRATORY DISORDERS

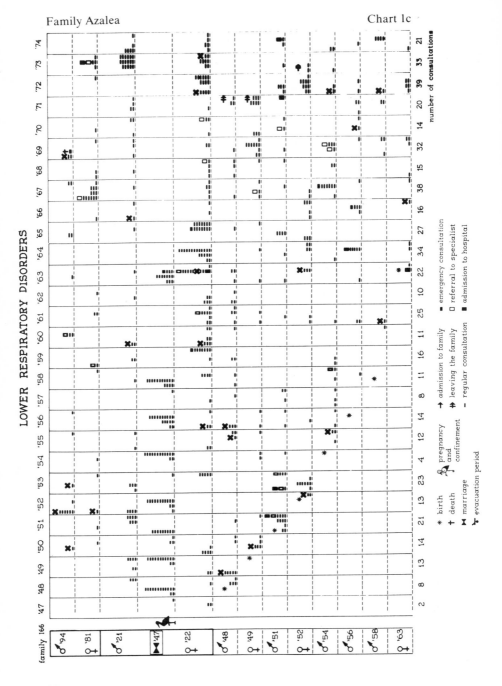

LOWER RESPIRATORY DISORDERS

Family Azalea

Chart 1c

168

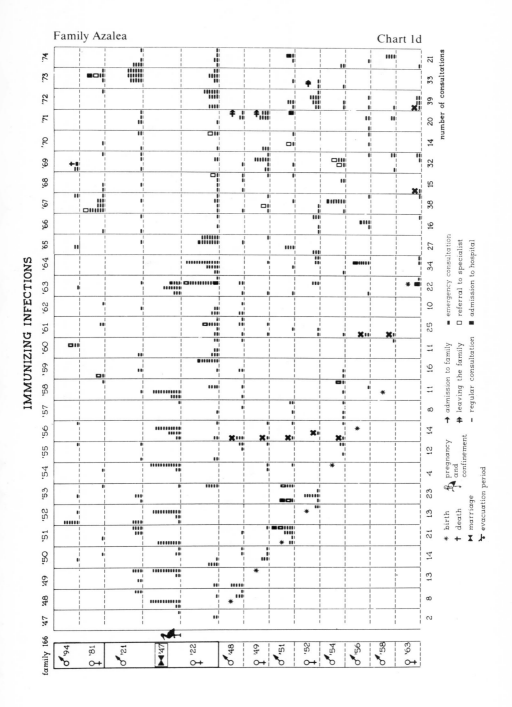

Family Azalea

Chart 1d

IMMUNIZING INFECTIONS

number of consultations

■ emergency consultation
↑ admission to family   □ referral to specialist
⇕ leaving the family   ■ admission to hospital
– regular consultation

* birth   ⚥ pregnancy
† death   and
✕ marriage   confinement
⚡ evacuation period

169

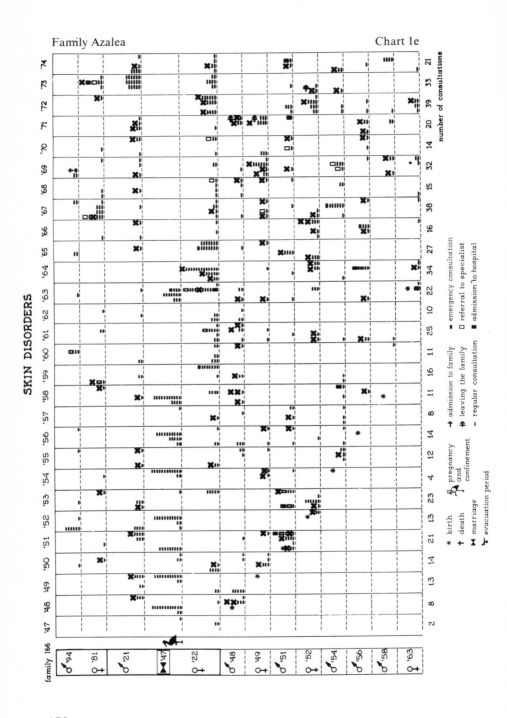

SKIN DISORDERS

Family Azalea   Chart 1e

170

GASTRO-INTESTINAL DISORDERS

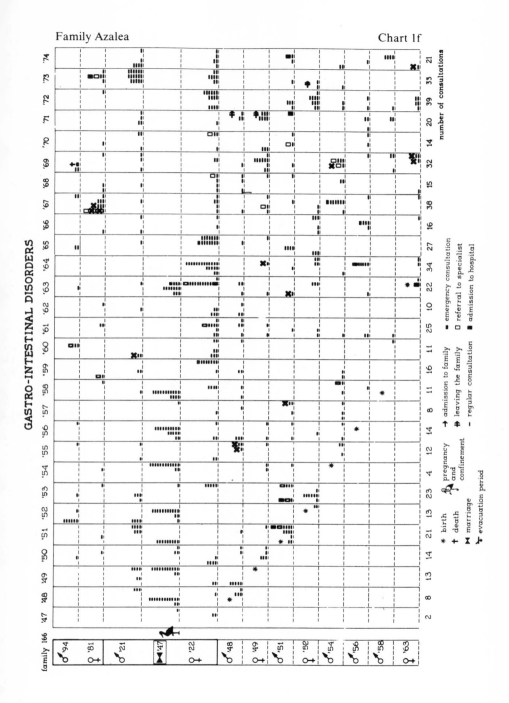

Family Azalea

Chart 1f

171

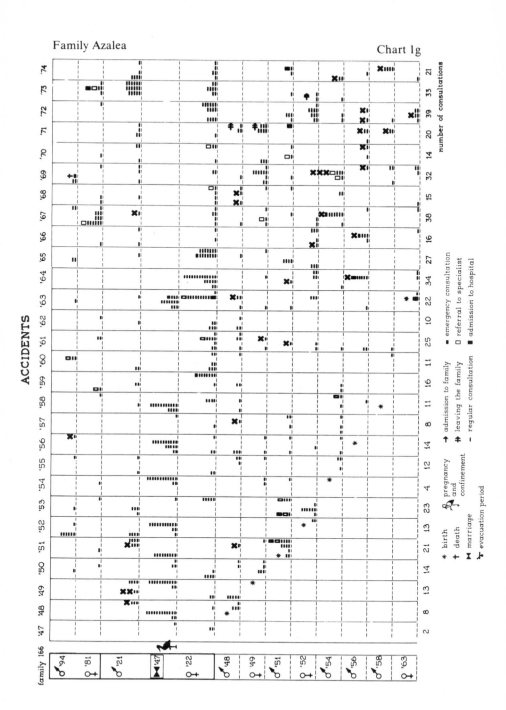

Family Azalea

Chart 1g

ACCIDENTS

172

NERVOUS DISORDERS

Family Azalea

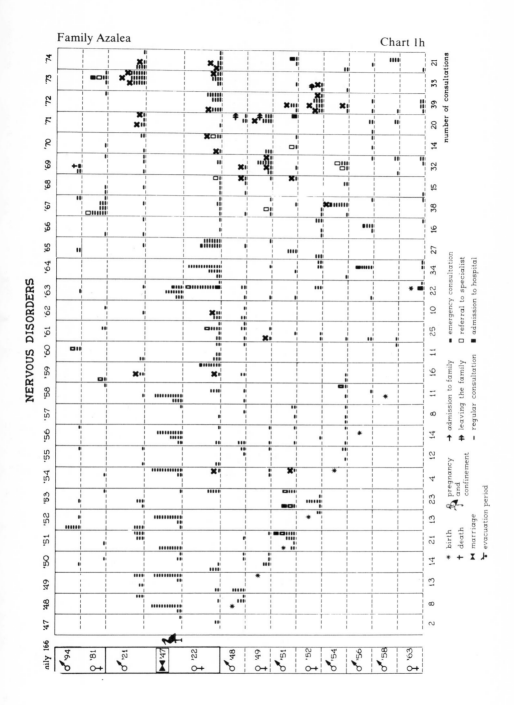

Chart 1h

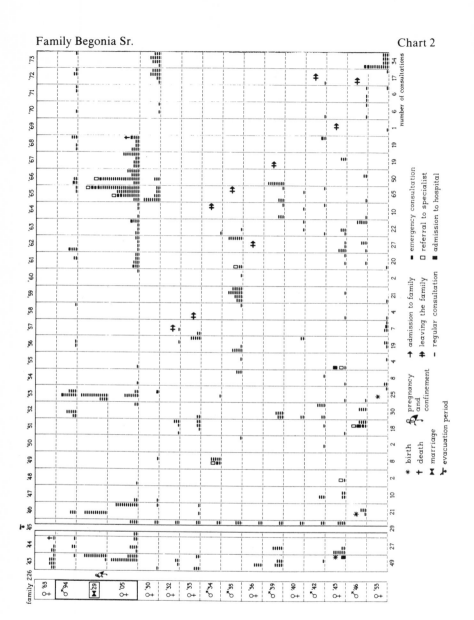

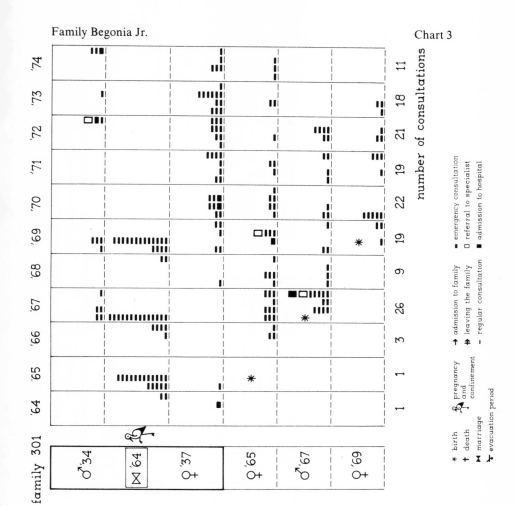

Family Begonia Jr.

Chart 3

number of consultations

family 301

* birth   ↑ admission to family   ■ emergency consultation
† death   ♠ leaving the family   □ referral to specialist
✗ marriage   – regular consultation   ■ admission to hospital
↳ evacuation period
♀ pregnancy and confinement

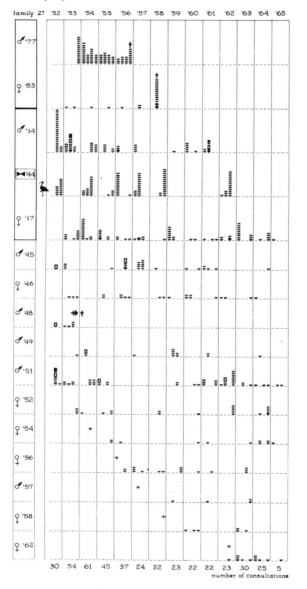

NERVOUS DISORDERS

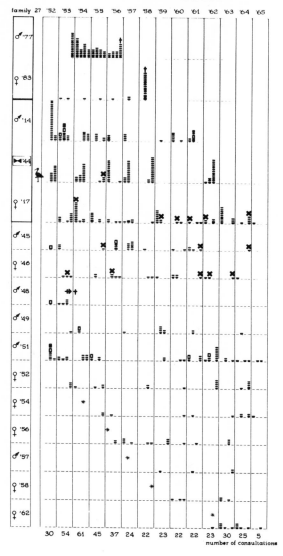

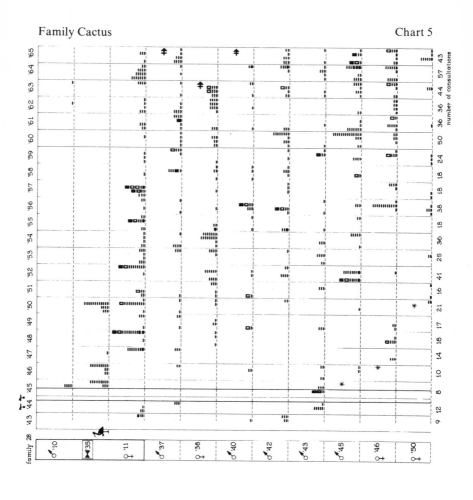

* birth   pregnancy   → admission to family   ▪ emergency consultation
† death   and confinement   ⊬ leaving the family   □ referral to specialist
⋈ marriage   − regular consultation   ▪ admission to hospital
⟙ evacuation period

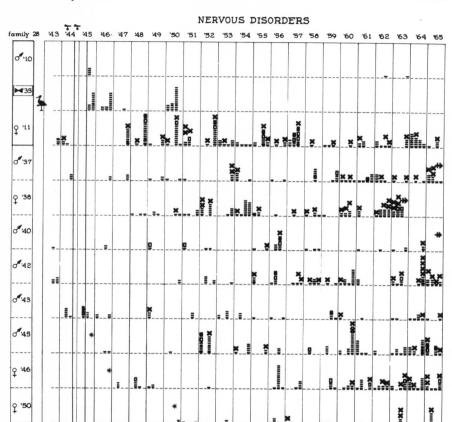

NERVOUS DISORDERS

NERVOUS DISORDERS

Chart 6

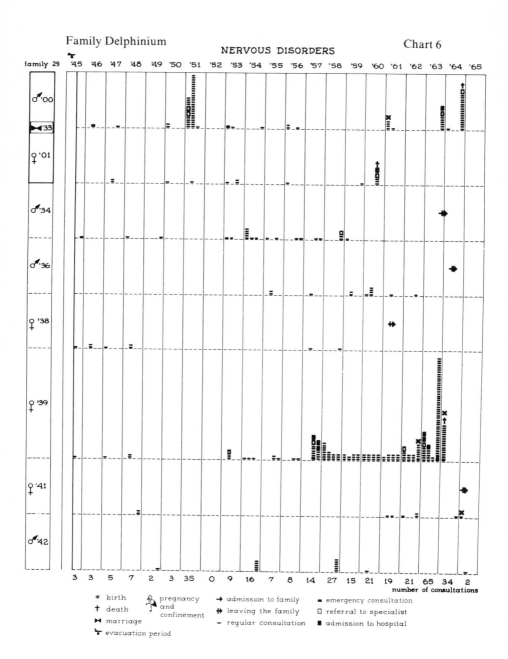

* birth
† death
⋈ marriage
⊤ evacuation period

🝆 pregnancy and confinement

→ admission to family
↠ leaving the family
− regular consultation

▪ emergency consultation
☐ referral to specialist
■ admission to hospital

number of consultations

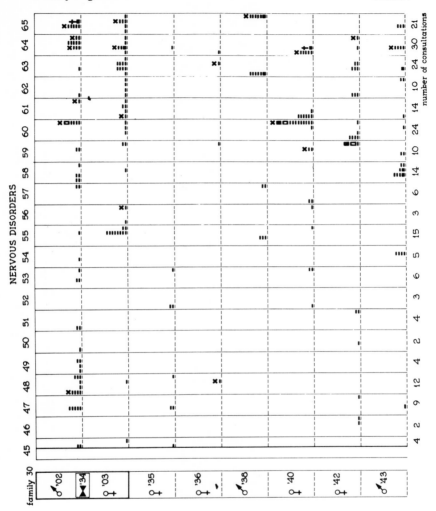

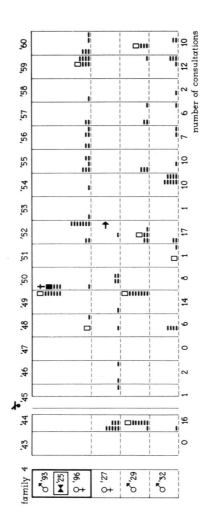

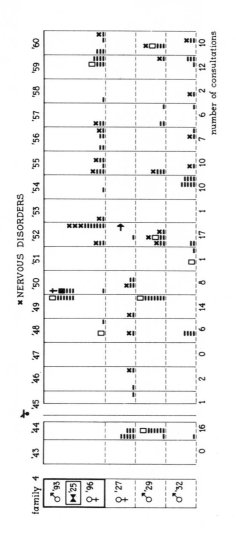

Chart 9

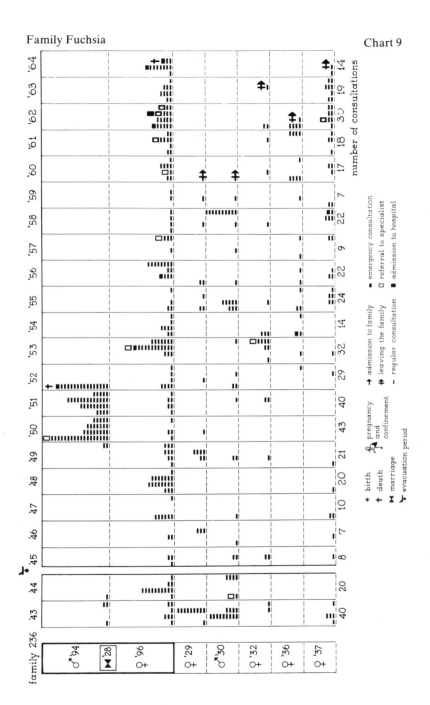

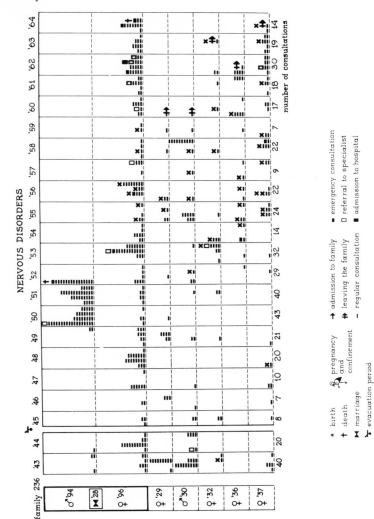

NERVOUS DISORDERS

number of consultations

* birth   pregnancy and confinement   ■ emergency consultation
+ death   confinement   □ referral to specialist
✗ marriage   ■ admission to hospital
⚓ evacuation period

* birth   ↑ admission to family   ■ emergency consultation
+ death   ⇞ leaving the family   □ referral to specialist
✗ marriage   – regular consultation   ■ admission to hospital
⚓ evacuation period

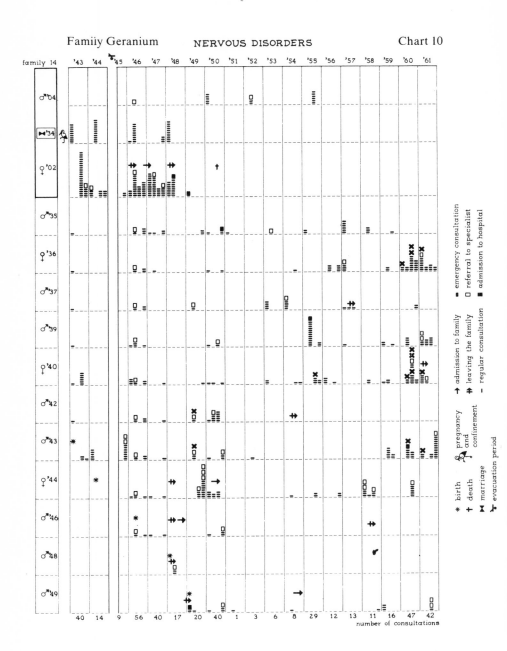

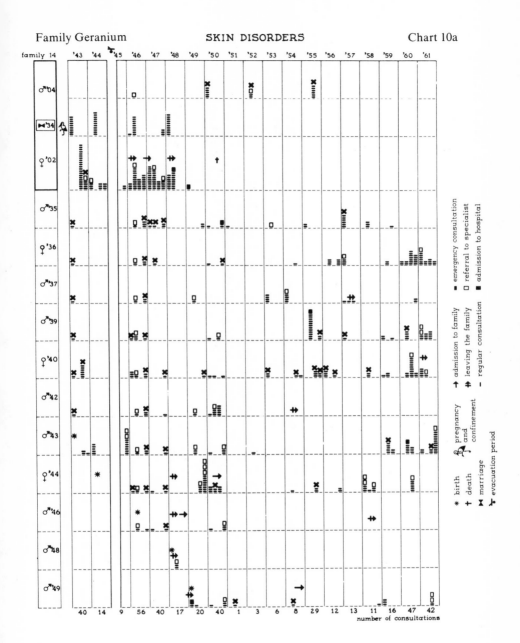

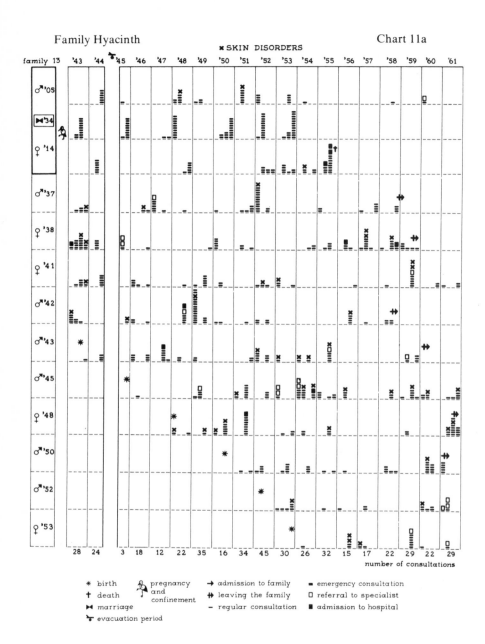

Family Hyacinth — Chart 11a

✻ SKIN DISORDERS

family 13   '43 '44 '45 '46 '47 '48 '49 '50 '51 '52 '53 '54 '55 '56 '57 '58 '59 '60 '61

number of consultations

28 24   3 18 12 22 35 16 34 45 30 26 32 15 17 22 29 22 29

✻ birth   pregnancy and confinement   → admission to family   – emergency consultation
† death   ⇥ leaving the family   ▢ referral to specialist
⋈ marriage   – regular consultation   ■ admission to hospital
⤙ evacuation period

188

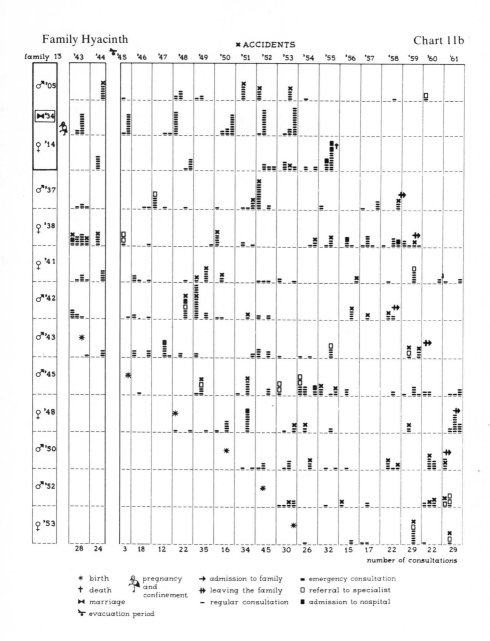

| family 13 | '43 | '44 | '45 | '46 | '47 | '48 | '49 | '50 | '51 | '52 | '53 | '54 | '55 | '56 | '57 | '58 | '59 | '60 | '61 |

number of consultations

28   24   3   18   12   22   35   16   34   45   30   26   32   15   17   22   29   22   29

* birth
† death
◄► marriage
⌐ evacuation period
pregnancy and confinement
→ admission to family
↟ leaving the family
– regular consultation
▪ emergency consultation
□ referral to specialist
▮ admission to hospital

189

Chart 12

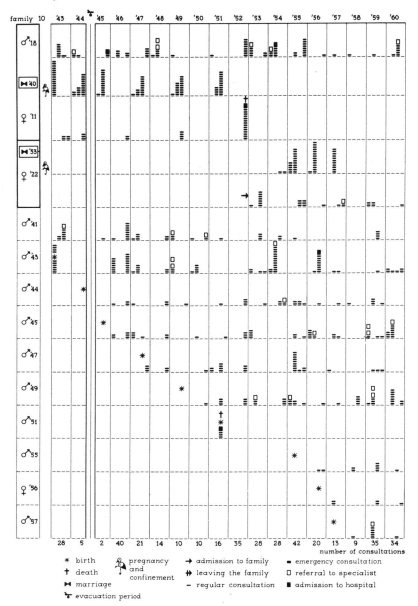

* birth
† death
⋈ marriage
⋎ evacuation period

🐦 pregnancy and confinement

→ admission to family
⇥ leaving the family
– regular consultation

▪ emergency consultation
□ referral to specialist
■ admission to hospital

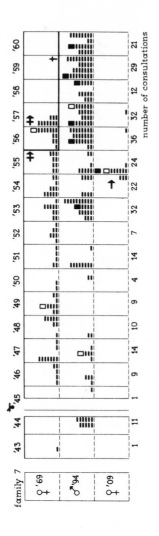

* birth   ℞ pregnancy   → admission to family   ▪ emergency consultation
† death   and   ⊬ leaving the family   □ referral to specialist
⋈ marriage   confinement   – regular consultation   ■ admission to hospital
⋏ evacuation period

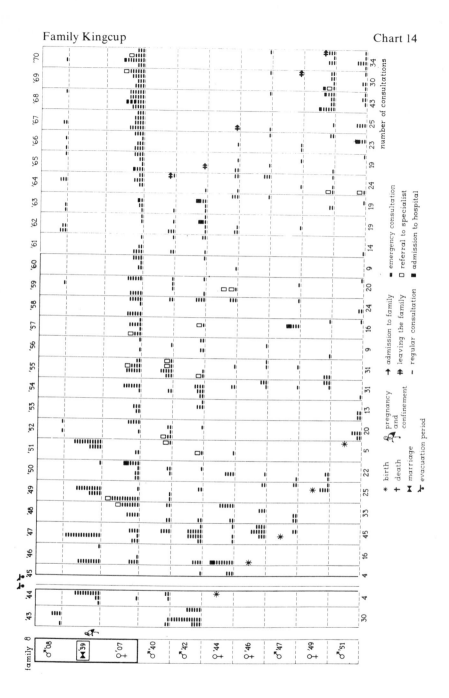

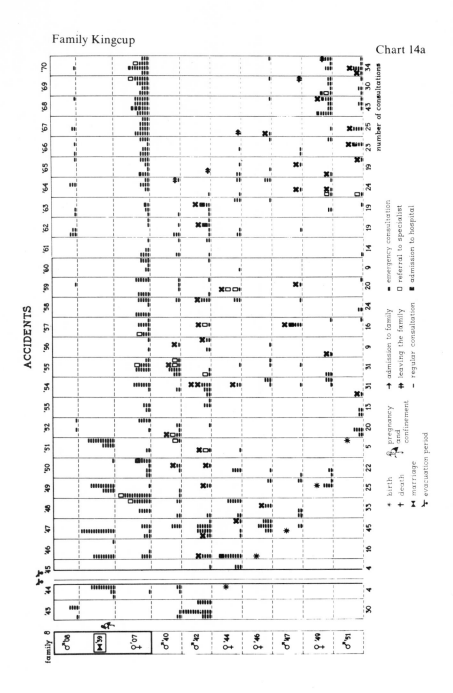

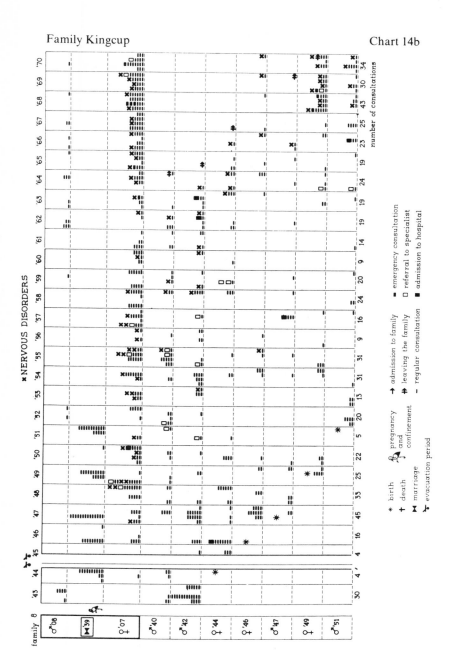

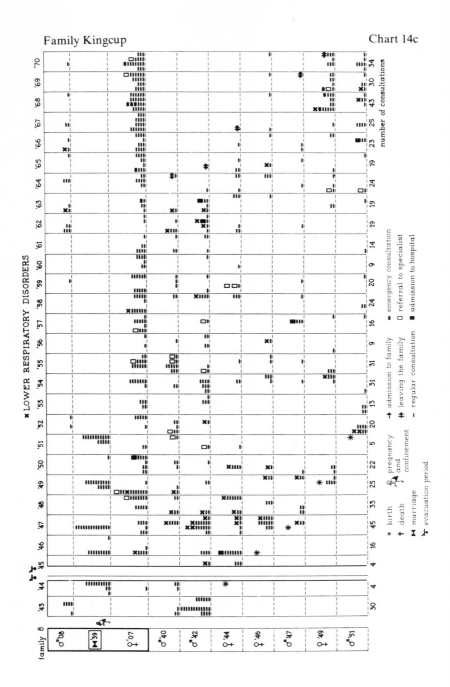

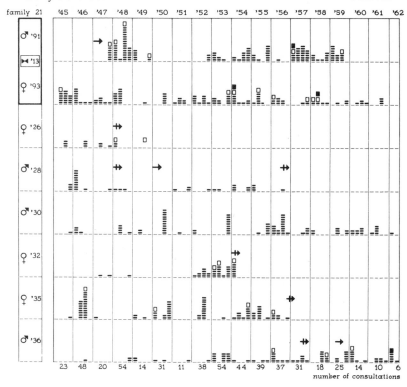

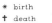

*	birth	♫	pregnancy	→	admission to family	▪	emergency consultation
†	death	♪	and confinement	✚	leaving the family	▫	referral to specialist
◄	marriage			–	regular consultation	■	admission to hospital
↧	evacuation period						

Family Lavender Jr.

Chart 16

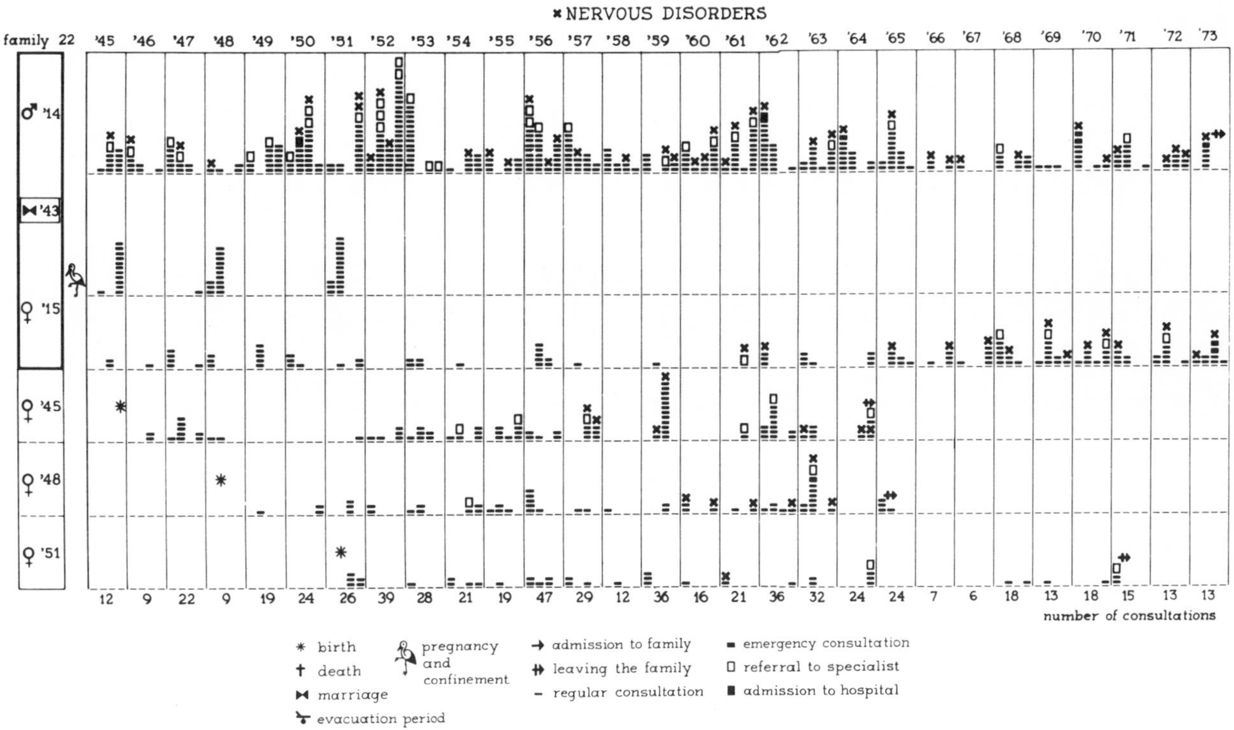
× NERVOUS DISORDERS
family 22
'45 '46 '47 '48 '49 '50 '51 '52 '53 '54 '55 '56 '57 '58 '59 '60 '61 '62 '63 '64 '65 '66 '67 '68 '69 '70 '71 '72 '73
♂ '14
⧓ '43
♀ '15
♀ '45
♀ '48
♀ '51
12 9 22 9 19 24 26 39 28 21 19 47 29 12 36 16 21 36 32 24 24 7 6 18 13 18 15 13 13
number of consultations
* birth
† death
⧓ marriage
evacuation period
pregnancy and confinement
→ admission to family
↛ leaving the family
- regular consultation
▪ emergency consultation
□ referral to specialist
■ admission to hospital

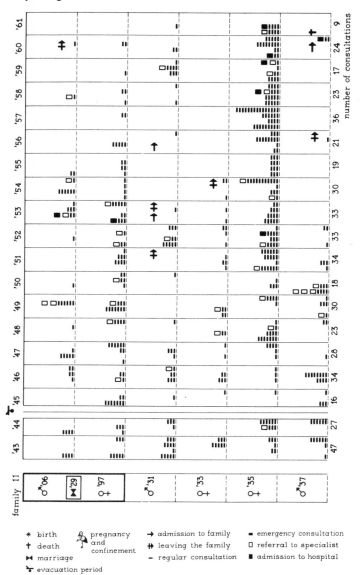

* birth   ♀ pregnancy   → admission to family   ■ emergency consultation
† death   and   ⇥ leaving the family   □ referral to specialist
⋈ marriage   confinement   – regular consultation   ■ admission to hospital
⤙ evacuation period

198

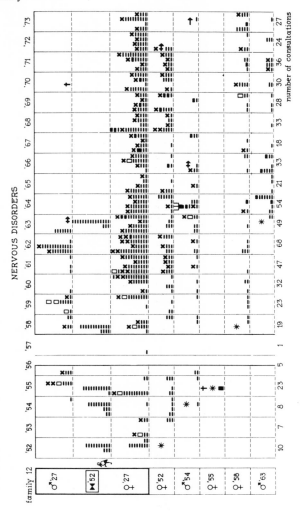

* birth   pregnancy   → admission to family   ▬ emergency consultation
† death   and   ⇥ leaving the family   ▢ referral to specialist
⋈ marriage   confinement – regular consultation   ▮ admission to hospital
⌄ evacuation period

199

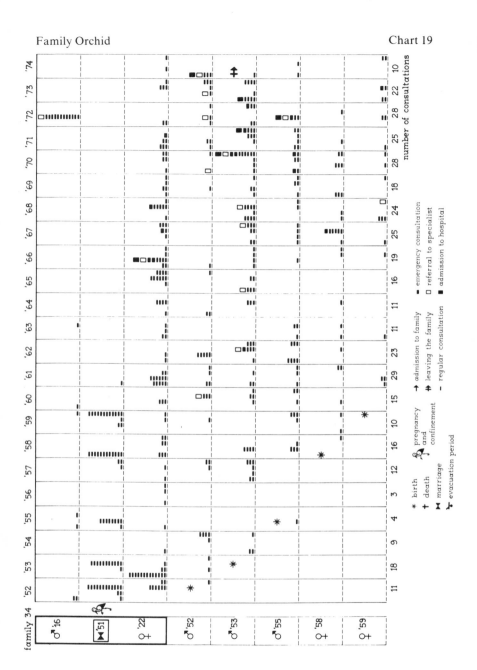

SKIN DISORDERS

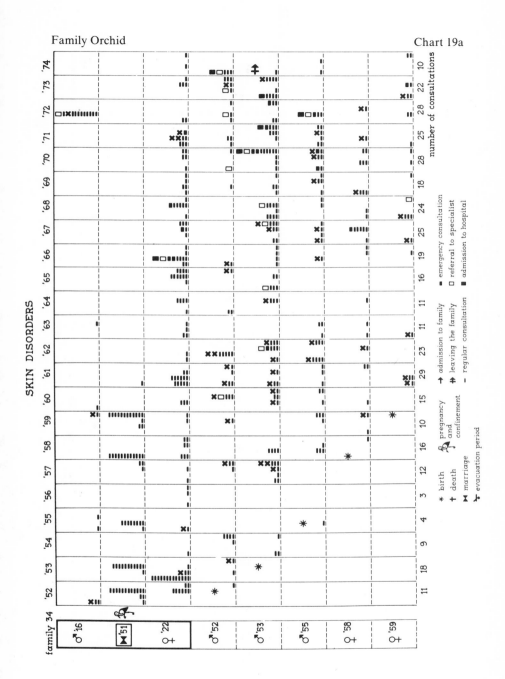

201

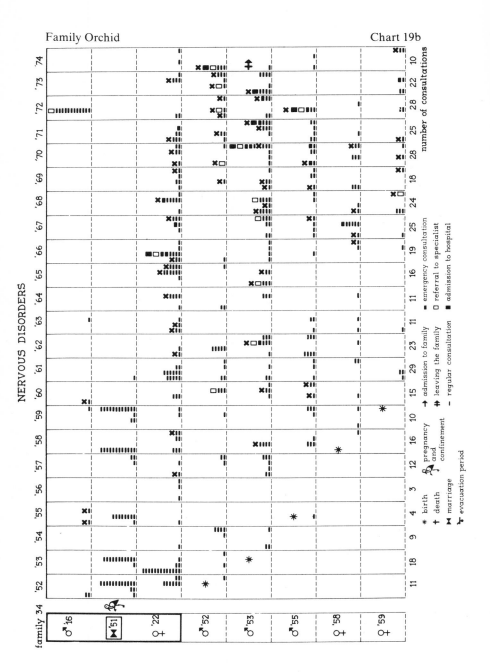

Family Orchid

Chart 19b

NERVOUS DISORDERS

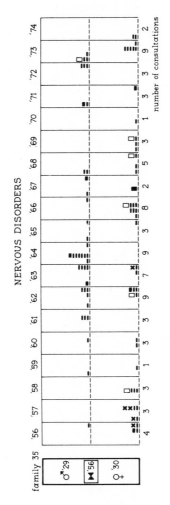

NERVOUS DISORDERS

NERVOUS DISORDERS

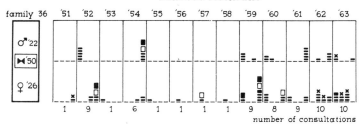

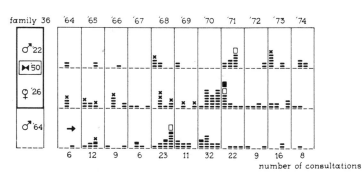

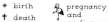

* birth
† death
⋈ marriage
☡ evacuation period

🦢 pregnancy
and
confinement

→ admission to family
⇾ leaving the family
− regular consultation

▬ emergency consultation
☐ referral to specialist
■ admission to hospital

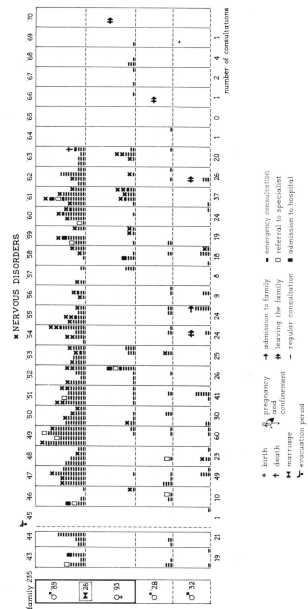

NERVOUS DISORDERS

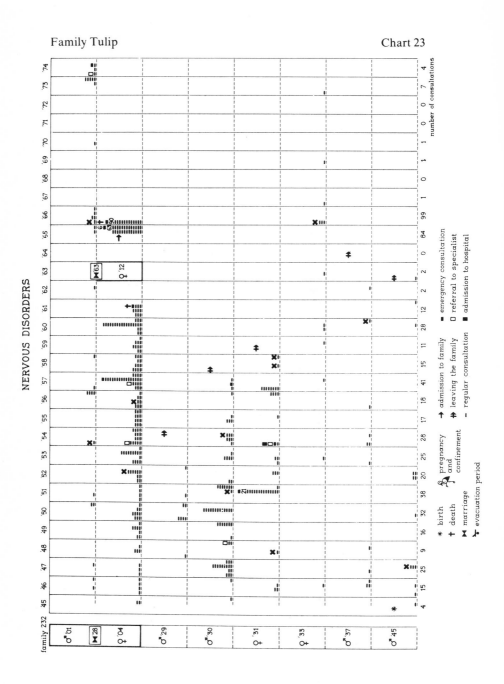

number of consultations

■ emergency consultation
□ referral to specialist
■ admission to hospital

↑ admission to family
↟ leaving the family
– regular consultation

⚥ pregnancy
   and
   confinement

∗ birth
† death
✗ marriage
⚚ evacuation period

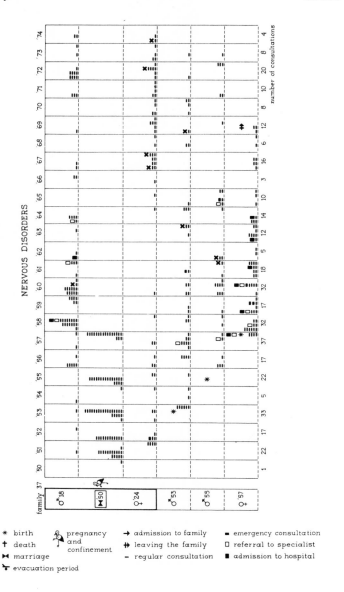

NERVOUS DISORDERS

* birth
† death
⋈ marriage
🔨 evacuation period

🦩 pregnancy and confinement

→ admission to family
⇥ leaving the family
– regular consultation

■ emergency consultation
◻ referral to specialist
▪ admission to hospital

Chart 25

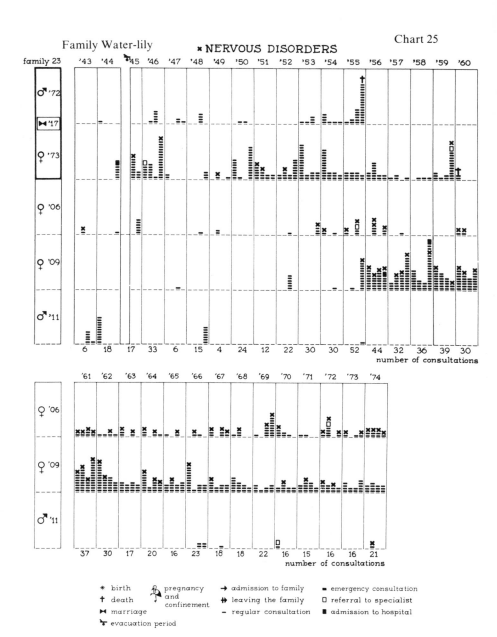

Family Water-lily ×NERVOUS DISORDERS

* birth
† death
◄ marriage
⸸ evacuation period

pregnancy and confinement

→ admission to family
↦ leaving the family
– regular consultation

▪ emergency consultation
□ referral to specialist
■ admission to hospital